I0022102

Defusing the Cancer Bomb

HOW CANCER SAVED MY LIFE

by Anna Gutkina

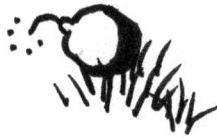

Illustrations by Curt Dilger

Illustrations - Curt Dilger
Book publication advice - Jill Cooper
Editor - Brittany Tobiason
Graphic design - Keith Fledderman
Chapter 19 illustration - Vitalia Golubovskaya
Chapter 20 illustration - Naomi Grigoryan
Chapter 23 illustration - Gary Welch

Copyright © 2014 Anna Gutkina
http://defusingcancerbomb.wordpress.com

All rights reserved. No part of this book may be
reproduced in any form or by any electronic or
mechanical means including information storage
and retrieval systems without permission in
writing from the author, except by a reviewer who
may quote brief passages in a review.

Some of the names and some of the details in this
narrative were altered to protect the integrity
of the story and to respect privacy of the people
associated with it.

⪢ GRATITUDE LIST ⪡

This book would not be possible without these people who supported the idea and me through the project. Without you this book would not exist. My gratitude goes to you:

Anton Mashanov and Alexey Wolfson for planting the idea of the book in my head.

Jill Cooper for her endless advice and encouragement in publishing this book.

Vitalia Golubovskaya for being my friend and believing in me as a scientist, an entrepreneur, and a writer.

Curt Dilger for making the illustrations and for having numerous conversations with me throughout the whole project .

Brittany Tobiason for being my editor.

Tatyana Ignatova for believing in me and for being an infinite source of ideas on how nature works in the darkness of time.

Alexander Grigoryan for support in raising our children and always providing me with food for thought, and Galina and Gevorg Grigoryan for helping out with the house work and the children while I was writing.

Olga Kotlovaya for the cheerful outlook, wit, encouragement and for sharing her fresh experience with publishing of her own book.

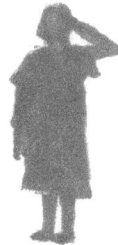

Betsy Kramer for running with me numerous miles for the cause of my book.

Jenkintown library for being my silent writer's refuge for hours.

Keith Fledderman for being creative, knowledgeable, and patient in putting this book together as a graphic designer.

All my dear friends who donated money and helped me paying for work on the book.

Without you this book would not exist.

TABLE OF CONTENTS

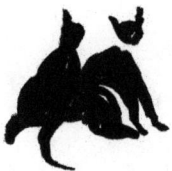

This book is dedicated to knowledge
and compassion acting in the world.
It was presented to me through my
family, my friends, and knowledgeable
and compassionate scientists and
doctors. This book is dedicated to active
knowledge and compassion in all of us.

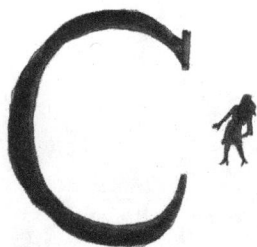

Foreword

Mine is a story of recovery from stage four peritoneal cancer via immunotherapy, a treatment with my own dendritic cells. When my life was extended far, far beyond my six month prognosis, I defused not only the cancer bomb, but some personal fate.

If you like suspense stories, personal narratives, silly important questions about death, love, marriage, creativity, gender riddles in Russia or whatever comes to mind while crossing borders, undergoing chemo or watching gondola makers, this story is also for you.

If you have a mind for business and think it could be your calling to make immunotherapy widely available and save more than just lucky over-educated, over-connected folk like me, this book is also for you. It explains something of the science behind my treatments.

But I wrote this book for my friend who feared for her life after her third cancer recurrence. I should have written it earlier and have wasted too much time, already. Skip those parts that you see as unnecessary sequins. Spend your time carefully and only on the relevant.

Prologue:
The Waiting Room

PATIENCE

You are waiting for your doctor's word and you are getting ready with your questions and with arguments that you carry from the internet, with friends' advice. Your arms are full of arguments. The waiting rooms are full of empty brochures. They say nothing about cures as you prepare your confrontational smile. The inappropriate laughter bombarding you from the TV is at jokes that might even be funny. I have compassion for anyone who has to watch sitcoms while preparing to hear what they can do to save their life. I sympathize with anyone who is sitting in a waiting room.

Even if the channel changes to the world news—all the fireworks of new federal elections, local killings, well-crafted speeches, arguments, hairdos, smiling heads, tanned and well presented—you remain languid, exigent, a world unto yourself, waiting for only one kind of news.

Before seeing the doctor, you will be weighed, your height measured. You will be asked to enumerate the glasses of wine you have consumed, the legal and illegal cigarettes. And if you say "None," the nurse with her clipboard will ask,"How about last year?" And if you still answer, "None," she will pursue you backward year by year to that half-pack a day habit when you were twenty two. A small voice in your head will start to guilt trip about all that wine, all those cigarettes. They become the possible reason why you are here bothering this doctor, who now seems as remote, as inaccessible, as great and powerful as the Wizard of OZ. The preparation could almost be intentional: a ceremony of distractions, a diversion thick as the stack of double-sided pages with tiny print that hangs, legal-sized, from the nurse's clipboard. By the time you are done answering questions, your mind is so numb, your confrontational smile so forgotten, he could tell you anything and you would not be able to find a single question among your arms, not an argument or even a thought.

When you do, finally, get your minute with the man, the myth, you will learn a problematic truth: every doctor is different. Some doctors will be aggravated with your faint attempts at logic, some not. Some doctors will be inclined to make you feel guilty for your illness. Some doctors will be patronizing. Some will give you false hope and make you numb to the urgency of treatment. Some will lie to you. Some will be very frank. Some will cry on your shoulder and say good bye.

You should expect to meet and assess a great many doctors and nurses to find a network of the best ones. This is the most urgent thing for you to do, now, while you are numbed by the irrelevant slack noise on the TV in the waiting room.

I know you might need some solutions right now and may be impatient for answers.

After giving you my recipe, I will go on and tell you the whole story of how I defused my cancer bomb.

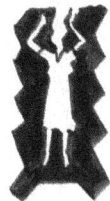

HUMILITY

Every time I sit in the waiting room to do my radiology exam, a blood test, or hear about results, I am very humble. No matter how confident I might seem between appointments—confident about my health and about how sensible my treatments are, and how joyous I am to still be alive—I am humble in anticipation of test results. I am humble going into the PET scan room, blood work lab, X-ray room, and later, sitting at the table in the doctor's office, and waiting for him to come in and announce my fate.

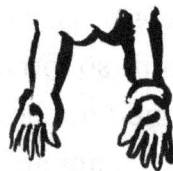

This is the room for shrinking and over-thinking. I panic and freeze, fearful of having done something to deserve a landslide back into disease. I go through all the slips in my diet, my sips of wine, my sins, my dreams, my children, my friends, my unfinished business. Was I too slow? Too stupid? I promise myself that if they declare that I am all right, I will be so very good: so strict with my diet and my care, spend so much time with my children and be so much more brilliant at work. Cancer demands humility. It drives a hard bargain.

Humility is why my book is not a celebration of my defeat of the beast of cancer. We are very vulnerable creatures, but there is a daring science that can cure us.

SLEEP

I always tried to resist the dreamy, noisy fog that makes us able to accept everything that we are told. Maybe I am not one of those non-feisty people who are okay with being numbed. I agree that I have always been an inconvenient presence in comfortable places. I agree, I may be an exception when I refuse to be cradled to sleep by the whole atmosphere of a hospital. I agree, I may be a crazy, rebellious Russian who is always ready for a fight. I accept that.

You should be a rebel too. There is an uncomfortable truth that sometimes a doctor does not know how to cure a patient. Sometimes, in a hospital, there is an acceptance of the immanence of death. Sometimes it is not justified. If there were no such acceptance, better practices would be in more common use.

The rhythmic dance between a doctor and a patient numbs both into mechanistic attitudes: so formal, so well-choreographed, so comforting. People who let themselves be soothed by the promises of doctors, such rhythmic promises—that everything is going to be okay, that they just have to have another round of chemo and radiation, that there is nothing to do but relax because they will be taken care of—they fall asleep in the wrong moment of their lives. They die very quickly.

Ignore the irrelevant and dreadful dream! Make a meaningful effort to have a second chance in life, a meaningful extension of your life! Wake up! Wake up!

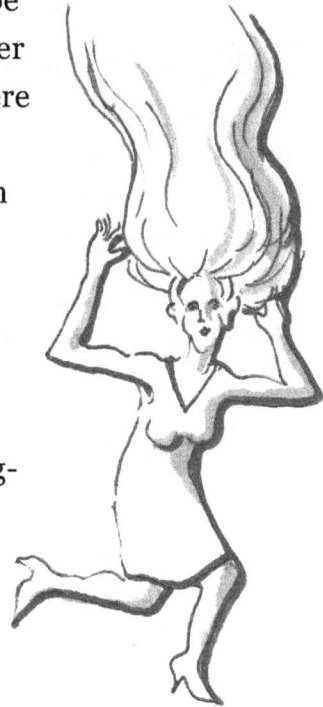

Introduction

=•=•=

WHAT TO DO IF YOU GET CANCER

Listen to those who know and trust them blindly. Don't listen to those who don't know. Skip their selfish advice. They just want to look helpful. Never spend your time doing research based on the flaky advice ignorant and careless people give you. They will tell you to research different options they just heard about—don't listen to them. Spend your time wisely. Listen to those "who were there" and survived. Make friends with them. Follow their directions. They know a lot of things that can make a life and death difference. They know the right people. They have proof to show. They are still "here."

At this moment in your life there is so much noise you have to ignore. And leave behind your worries! You will get to them later.

Surgery and chemotherapy are the standard treatments any doctor is likely to recommend. It is common knowledge that this combination is not a cure. Find the best doctors you

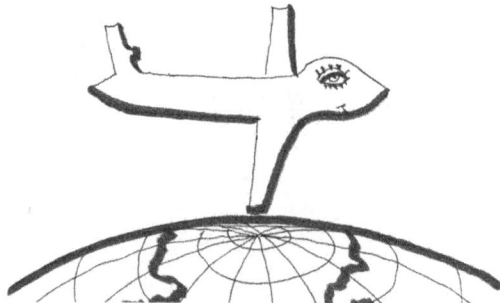

can and get second and third opinions, every time. If you have a bad feeling or your treatment doesn't seem right, trust that feeling. Seek personal care.

· I ·

If you are extremely lucky, your doctor will perform immunotherapy, which will train your immune system to attack cancer cells anywhere in your body. Immunotherapy treatment begins with a surgery to remove the tumor. The cells of the tumor are then used to create a dendritic cell vaccine.

Your treatment should also include an anti-metastatic vaccine to target future metastases. Ninety percent of deaths from cancer occur from metastases, which are the growths of multiple tumors from sleeper cells. The main tumor is always shedding cells. These circulate in the body, dividing to multiply. When under attack by treatments such as chemotherapy, that target dividing cells, roaming cancer cells temporarily stop dividing. They "hide" in a state of dormancy. It is necessary to eradicate these sleeper cells that cause metastasis.

I am alive because of immunotherapy. I experienced no side effects.

· II ·

I tried a lot of things. I don't know which of them worked. In retrospect, I was my own guinea pig. Some things I did based on specific information, some I did blindly. But before the question "why" is answered, all I can say: this is what I did, and it's your choice to justify or not justify, analyze or not analyze, to do the same things or not to do, but here they are:

a) Sodium butyrate - I still take 10 mg per day, even now, four years after the diagnosis. Whenever I have discontinued it, I have gotten nervous. Sodium butyrate is thought to unpack the DNA of certain genes and make it available for the cellular machinery that synthesizes important anti-cancerous proteins. These proteins are the foundation of strictly balanced cell health.

b) Macrobiotic diet - You should find a nutritionist that can provide good guidance .Carrot juice: two to three glasses a day.

c) If you do decide to include chemotherapy among your treatments, there are herbs that can be prescribed for you by any practitioner of traditional Chinese medicine.

d) Aspirin - Daily aspirin will prevent clotting and inflammation, both known to cause errors in cellular development and to cause cancer.

e) Meditation - a sit in a group once a week, or 108 meditative breaths every day. Make it a 100 breaths rule. You will connect to yourself, a strange quiet being inside of your skin, somewhere in your lower belly, where it's dark and peaceful.

f) Do the things now that you want to be alive for - Fill your life with joy in any way you can.

I am writing this in an Italian bistro in Lipari, a small island where people live so close to their gods that everything feels tranquil and meaningful. These are called the Aeolian Islands, in the name of Eol, a god of breath. I am breathing in and out, in and out: the sea breeze, the view, the life, here, in Lipari. Four years ago, I was not sure I would be here on Earth, especially on this wonderful mythical island. But here I am, completely alive.

TRUST

Today, I look back on those days of distress: the sweaty, sleepless nights, the endless phone calls, fear of the end, the solitude of desperation, and know that I was going to survive. I did not know then, that loving friends would defuse my distress and sadness and solitude and shame. I did not know that brilliant scientists would cure my cancer. I did not know that I would have to travel to find the answer that was immunotherapy treatment in Russia. I did not know that it would take so many inexplicable, serendipitous events to concoct the vaccine that would cure my cancer.

In retrospect, events unraveled magically. However, when I was in the midst of it, while I was doing my treatments and travels, it felt like a disaster. I really had no time do anything but react. I was receiving a lot of different advice and trying to take it all. I was never sure I was doing the right thing.

The traditional treatment was chemo-therapy. Scientist friends who survived cancer by immunotherapy alone warned

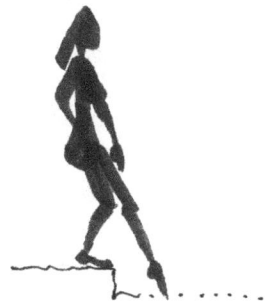

me against chemotherapy. But, two other scientists friends refused chemotherapy and died from cancer. I chose to try it, but didn't know if I'd done the right thing by starting chemotherapy.

I understand how lucky I am. Being originally from Russia, going there for treatment was easy. I just stayed at my parents' house. It was like going home. I am also a biologist, so the science of it all made sense to me. I am known here in Philadelphia as a "miracle neighbor." We know my recovery is due to science, but I also had to trust strangers, take chances and decide to do whatever it took. My heart bleeds for all those who have died because they were too afraid to trust, too afraid to risk, too afraid to fight for their lives.

Most cancer patients who ask me what they should do are not biologists, and most of them are not Russian. When I urge them, as I was urged, to go to Russia for immunotherapy, they are facing a much more difficult decision than I faced. They never go to Russia, and they never look for immunotherapy in the US either. How many more lives will be saved, each year, when the treatment that cured me is considered standard practice?

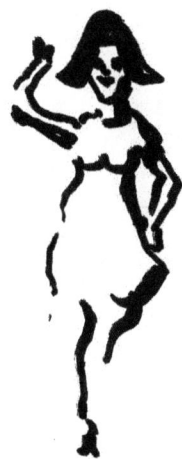

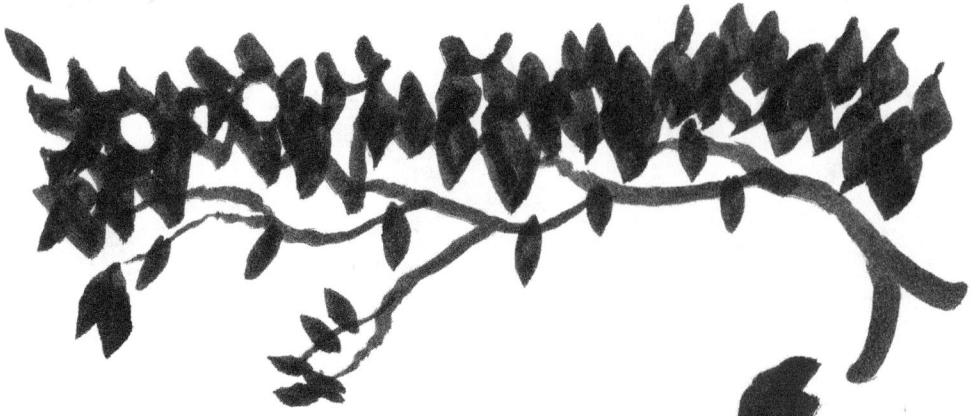

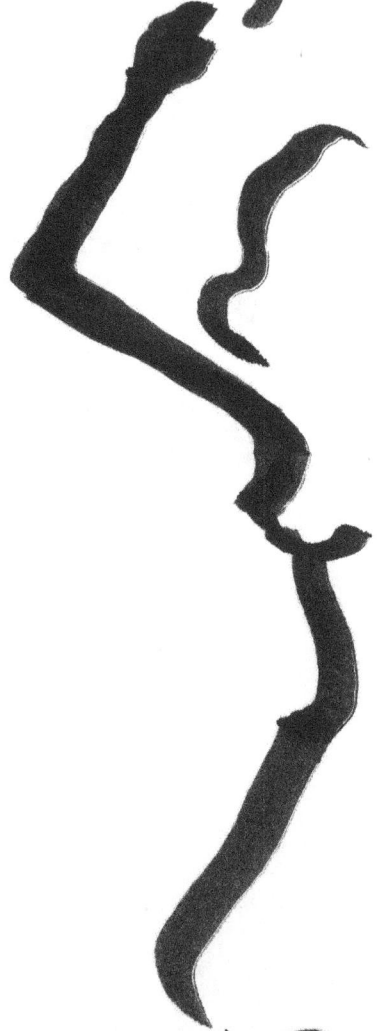

PART I

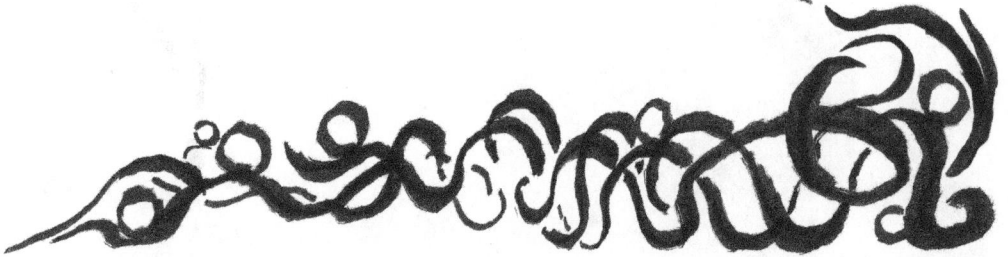

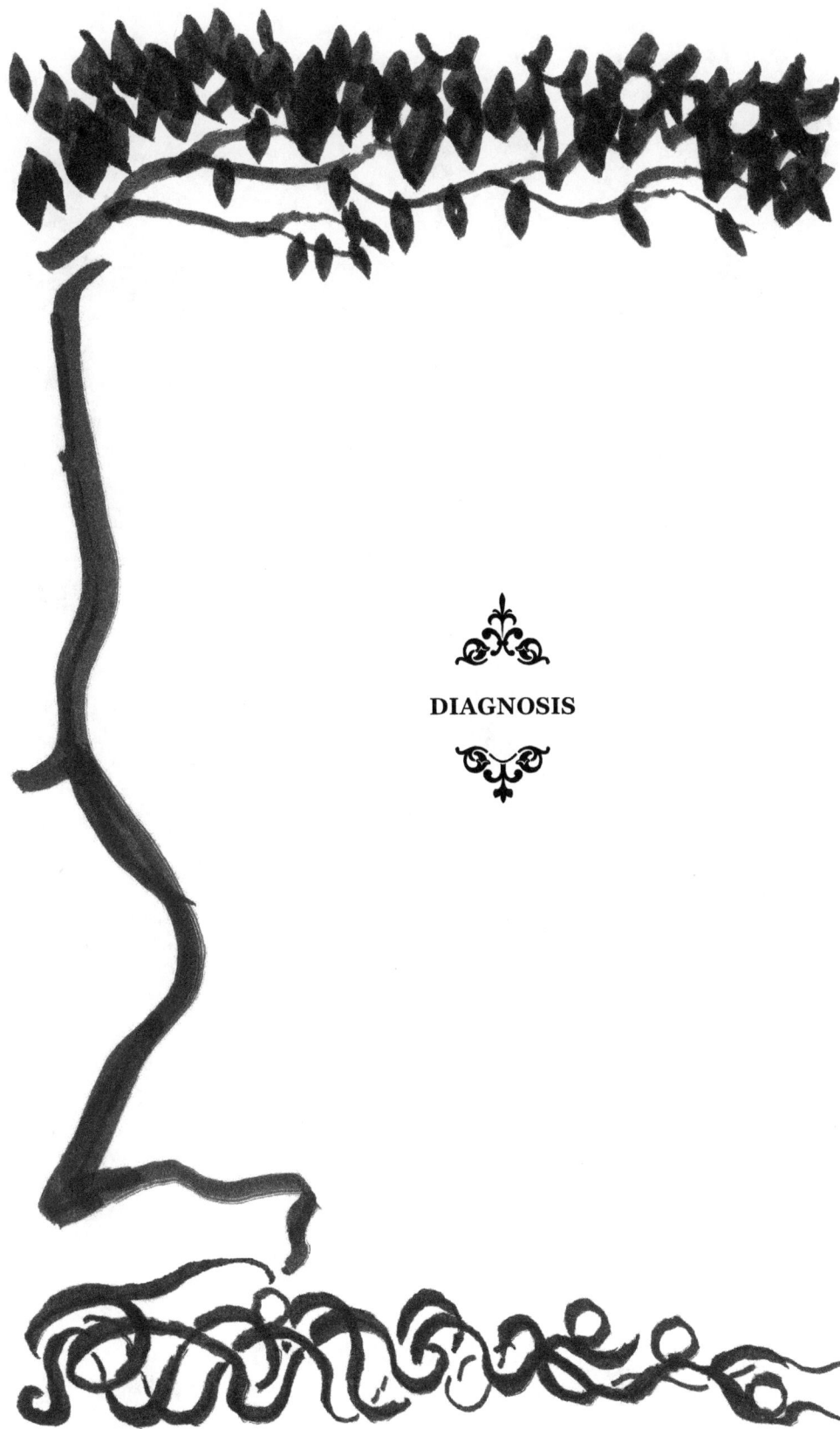

DIAGNOSIS

CHAPTER 1
Silence

✦ I ✦

One morning, I lost my speech. Let's start with this. One morning, I felt so incredibly sick that I began vomiting. I had to wait for my husband, Gosha, to come back from work to go to the emergency room. He wasn't sure I wasn't making it up but, finally, he agreed and we drove to the nearby hospital's Emergency Room. There, after waiting in the usual line, we were greeted by a joyful doctor, joking and taking it easy. Kidding and teasing, he made an X-Ray of my lungs and sent me home with the prescription for an antibiotic. "Pneumonia," he said.

I took the antibiotic and, by morning, my vomiting went away. Gosha left for work. I stayed home to finally sleep and start to recover. In the late morning, my cell phone rang. I barely opened my eyes, reached for the phone but, when I opened my mouth, I found I could not make a sentence. I somehow pushed out a, "Hi." The caller, a new acquaintance from a business networking meeting, started talking but all I could think of was how terrifyingly hard it had been to speak. I said something short like, "Sorry, I am busy now." I had to hang up. Something was very wrong. I tried to keep talking to myself just to test it. It was getting worse and worse. I sent my husband an email to come home as soon as he could. He did not believe me. He waited till the end of his business day. "Honey, you are exaggerating," he sighed.

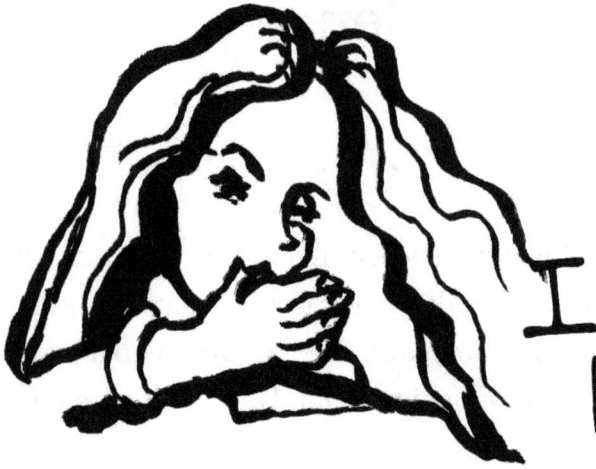

I had
to
watch

I had to watch my speech deteriorate until
he came home. I now was so devastated and
confused that I gave up fighting and just waited for him to
come home and take care of me. I just hoped he would take
me to the ER again. I could not even argue with him as, by
evening, I had lost all of my ability to speak. I don't remember if he tried to make fun of the situation. I think he did
make some jokes at the emergency room when they were
asking the routine questions that I had learned by heart
but no longer could answer: What is your name? What is
your date of birth? He had to answer for me. It could have
been defensive laughter, but I remember vividly that Gosha
sort of giggled when we met the joking doctor from the day
before and told him we were back but with the difference
that I could no longer speak.

✦ II ✦

Waiting.Waiting.In the waiting room.Receptionists.

"My wife can't talk and she is vomiting."

"Are you her husband? Take a seat. You will be called."

Did someone ask me to step onto the scale? I don't remember. Had there been a wheel chair? Perhaps they took my temperature. Then, we were closed into a room.

A long time passed. Gosha would peek out of the room from time to time to look for someone in charge. Perhaps a nurse came. Perhaps more than once. Eventually, yesterday's joking doctor came in and started to ask me questions. "She can't talk," Gosha said with a hint of a giggle. I tried to say my name but could not and gave up. "What is your name?" the joking doctor asked. "She can't talk." I felt really miserable and from then on I stopped even trying. I could still write at this point and I was trying to write something, however later I wouldn't be able to do that, either. Only then did I begin to really notice how many times a patient is asked by numerous people at a hospital his name and date of birth. I don't remember if I came up with any system of answering. I think I just didn't answer. I think I just sat in that embarrassing, humiliating wheelchair. I think I just lay on that bed:

my speech deteriorat e

so vulnerable, so at the mercy of anyone's eyes, further weakened by my husband's smirking suspicions.

"Can't talk?" The no-longer-laughing doctor finally believed my husband.

He disappeared. I saw him again four years later, when he walked into a Starbucks where I was writing this book, even while I was writing this chapter. But that was the only other time I ever saw him.

A new doctor came in and announced that he would be in charge. He had an expression of thoughtful concentration over the tough case that I was. He focused on doing tests quickly, one after another. I was rushed to different test stations and test machines. He was not joking. He was different from the rest of the habitually overconfident and mandatorily brash doctors of the emergency room. He had a combination of a usual aloofness and an intense attention; no patting on the back in a manner intended to remind one of a beer buddy, a chum, a friend from childhood. His thoughtfulness and slowness made him look somewhat provincial in the shiny environment of the emergency room made dramatic by association with Emergency Room TV. I refer to him here as Doctor Slow. He did not fall into the other category of doctor either, the one most East Indian doctors seemed to belong to, especially in the beginning of their American careers. Perhaps because they did not watch much television, these doctors were not chic but rather pompous, bellied, and all together godly, still carrying the weight that Indian culture puts on the figure of Medical Doctor. It was with this second type that I would have the most problems, as I was about to find out in my

Hospital Odyssey.

My Slow and Thoughtful Doctor was not a typical emergency room doctor, and I realized that in his profession some general slowness might mean thoughtfulness and proficiency. Slowly but surely.

Doctor Slow started to get to the bottom of my speechlessness and nausea. He ordered an MRI brain scan. The results showed multiple infarcts or clots in my brain. In both hemispheres.

"WHAT??? Infarcts?Multiple?In both hemispheres?" Gosha was lost.

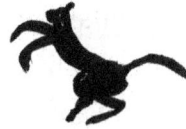

"It means she had a stroke."

I heard everything but could not say anything, could not ask the strings of questions that usually made Gosha so self-conscious, so ashamed of me. Now he was ashamed by the fact that I had had a stroke. I was ashamed too. It is part of our culture, to be always strong and winning. Disease is perceived as a sign of weakness. We were both the children of tough Russian culture.

Perhaps I was not as horrified as Gosha because I had just read a book about strokes. It was a recent release and a common topic of discussion. I peeked at it when I got it. Oh God, I just realized I still have the book, never returned it! Did you notice that if a book is not returned it starts a life in your life? It was *The Stroke of Insight* by Jill Bolte Taylor. She had suffered a terrible stroke in which her left hemisphere was almost shut off. She lost her speech too and was in a horrible state, perhaps worse than mine. She recovered, and her fantastic book is the account of her experience. I had recently had discussions about her accurate and detailed description of what it is like to have your mind shut down all logic and language and give in to the pleasures of the intuitive, visual, creative right hemisphere.

The fact that somebody went through the stroke before me and had recovered was, at that point, all the reassurance I needed. Reminiscing about the neighbor's party, at which I'd had such a lively discussion about this book, effectively smoothed the rough shock of the news. Familiarity with a subject takes away the horror of the unknown. I found myself even a little excited that relearning how to speak might be a way to get rid of my Russian accent! Can you believe that?

Although Doctor Slow did not quite answer Gosha's questions about how there came to be multiple infarcts in my brain, he did one tremendously important thing: he started to give me anti-clotting injections. He hooked me to a bag with heparin solution. I think he deliberated about the exact concentration of it, given that there would be no personnel over the weekend to watch me. From then on it would be constant blood work.

Over the weekend, Gosha brought friends to visit me in my room at Hope Memorial Medical Center. Gosha's friend Roma came to visit with his children in tow and, later, a friend who is a physical therapist came, too. I did not even pretend to welcome them but, since I could not speak and they did not even notice my embarrassment, I just sat there almost crying while Roma stayed in my room, smiling and disciplining his kids. He stayed a long time to be polite, and it was way too long for me. Why did all these friends of Gosha's have to come?!

I did not think at the time that I was lucky. It all developed so quickly. Monday came and went and they still were taking blood samples. Gosha's friend, Dr. Tolik was constantly on the phone with him, interpreting the blood tests. They talked for hours on end about the coagulation. Nobody could tell why my coagulation was so high.

All the doctors from my Family Doctor's office where well known on this floor, accommodating mostly long time retirees, who were sometimes very sad shells of patients. I suspect Hope Memorial's office supervised a nursing home. These patients were mostly very weak and usually bed ridden. They never left their rooms. If they asked, it was an emergency. Otherwise, they were just there, barely present, and totally dependent on the system for every breath.

✦ III ✦

It is a dream. No. It's not. Every morning I go through a visitation by a procession of doctors and interns. They listen to the lead doctor and write on their clipboards.

"She is speechless," he explains. "Oh, what is your name?" they ask. I wave and look at them in humiliation. "See?" And the whole procession moves on. *But what about me? Come back! Tell me why I had a stroke! But they are always already gone.*

This was waking life. During their morning routine, the

doctors and nurses would pinch off enough time to ask: "And how are you doing Ms. Gutkina?" But by the time I opened my mouth, still unable to speak, they were gone. Their miniscule quotas of attention, their precisely throttled routes, their internal needs: all made them completely oblivious to the environment. An environment of introverted people, silent, passive, parchment bodies— made ghostly by design of the system that promised to heal them—glided by and around me like clouds.

I had expected to be cared for in the hospital. I had expected people to know I had to survive to raise my children. I had expected someone to try do something out of the ordinary to save my life. I noticed I was being avoided. I started to realize that remaining silent would kill me

**DEDICATION &
CERTIFICATION OF
THANKS TO:**

*Lynn, Joe,
Tora, Ella, and
Seth Pokrifka*

**ANNA THANKS YOU FOR
YOUR KIND SUPPORT!**

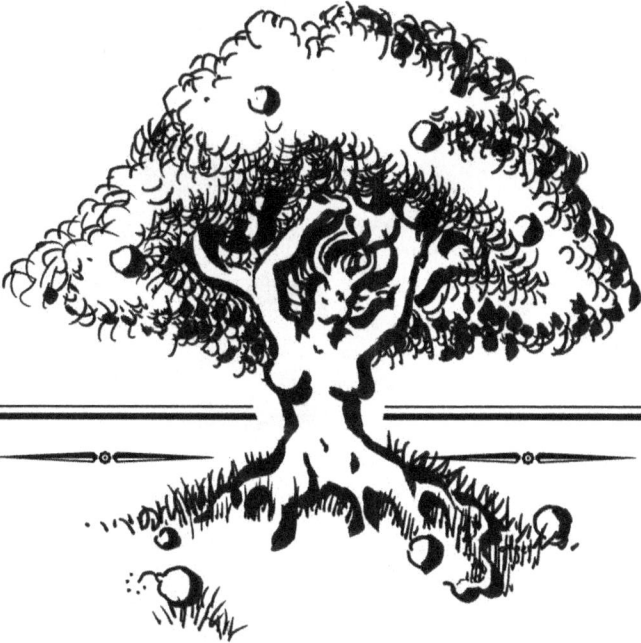

CHAPTER 2
The Swollen Legs

Eventually, it was discovered that my stroke had been caused by clots in my legs that had gone undetected and traveled to my brain. "Undetected" is not quite the right way to put it. This is the real beginning of my story.

∽ I ∽

It was winter in Philly, white and early. I was at the end of my MBA studies, taking a class. I felt awful. I usually like snow, especially the first light, puffy, calm snowflakes, but that day I barely noticed it. My feet dragged disturbingly slowly on the ground, as I walked very slowly from my car, unable to keep up with a friend because I had so much pain and stiffness in my legs. When he gave me a surprised look, I realized that my condition might really be as awful as it felt. I could barely sit in the accounting class that seemed endless. I felt sick in the stomach, just unusually sick. And my legs ached.

At some point I started to complain about the leg pain to my shrink. "Yes," she said, "It's because you don't know where to go in life." She was an adamant believer in the psychosomatic manifestation of emotional issues in the body. For every ailment there would be a psychological explanation. I believed it too. However, the pain was becoming unbearable, especially at night. I would wake up with throbbing legs and want to cry. Finally, I went to see a family doctor. I requested an appointment with the head of the practice, Dr. Weldon K. Moore, but he didn't have an opening until July.

I had already met and did not want to see the available Dr. Blavatkez, who worked under Dr. Moore in the same office. He never sounded knowledgeable and looked like law suit material to me. I went to see him anyway. "Let's make sure it is not this," he named something very rare and exotic, looking things up in his lap top. He ordered a test for this rare disease that I was not likely to have. "We're just making sure," he assured me and called for his nurse to take my blood. A young male nurse appeared, iridescent with the self-importance and capricious playfulness of an actor playing the role of a nurse. He was armed with a needle and stuck it into my veins several times without success. He tried and tried. When it became ridiculous, I told him I had had enough. I asked him to go away and send someone who knew what they were doing. The little page was upset and let me hear his raspy complaints to somebody in the inner chambers of Dr. Moore's office.

After a while another nurse came in. "How are you Ms. Gutkina? Are we taking some blood today?" After this perfunctory polite exchange, she took my blood successfully. I was also scheduled for ultrasound scans of my legs to be done in three weeks.

"Three weeks," I asked? "I am in pain right now."

"I cannot do anything, Ms. Gutkina. I am sorry. It is either three weeks or no test. It is up to you."

"Can't you call them and say it is an emergency?"

"Ms. Gutkina, I am working hard here. I told you already. Come back in three weeks," insisted Dr. Blavatkez

"But you said we need to eliminate the possibility of blood clots. Is that not urgent?"

"This is to make sure you don't have them, which is very likely. If it were a clot it would have been in one leg, not in both legs. Plus, you are too young to have clots. Plus, I am working hard here, Ms. Gutkina." He went back into the office and had another conversation with Dr. Moore. "Nope. Sorry. Bye-bye, Ms. Gutkina."

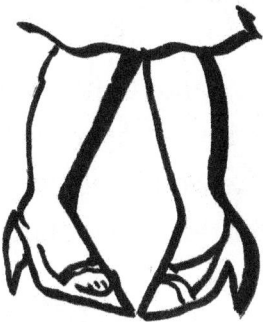

At that time, I was just a provincial virgin of a patient. I did not know yet, then, that I should not have taken their pompous scheduling problems for an answer. During the major medical journey that was about to start, I would meet with doctors who would have made sure I was connected with the right specialist immediately, right that day, right that hour. They would have picked up a phone. Well, at that deeply unfortunate time, I was shy and naïve, sitting with my dumb, sad face and huge problem. In pain, in the stupid suburban office, at the mercy of its masters, I was lost, defeated and I didn't know where to turn.

∞ II ∞

After three weeks of awful pain in my legs, I came to see a
technician at the local suburban hospital that had a special
facility for ultrasound examinations, to look for clots in my
legs. The technician had the same Russian-Ashkenazi blue
eyes, wavy dark hair, and pale skin that I do. She might
have been brought to America by her family as a child.
She did not have an accent. I felt her animosity right off
the bat. I felt it very strongly, unusually strongly. I could
never explain it well to my American friends but, when two
Russians in America meet for the first time, they don't like
each other. They actually almost hate each other. There is
intense competition and jealousy. We would assess each
other's class via the usual status symbols of money, car and
job. Seeing a different version of the self, with a different
fate, always inspired a strong mix of feelings about one's
own success. Perhaps I seemed to outclass my younger twin
and this was disturbing for her. Perhaps she wondered what
I filled my days with while she had to suffer through looking
at other people's deep vein thrombosis.

I had learned to recognize and overcome it
in myself, but it was clear to me that this girl
had not, that I was disturbing to her. She
glared at me with extreme hostility. I tried to
sweeten up the conversation with jokes. I asked
her friendly questions. She stared at me and
muttered something in response while starting
the ultrasound machine. The technician maintained an
expression of vaguely vengeful resentment and disgust. I
could not see the screen at which she was staring.

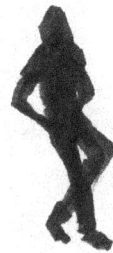

"So? I asked. Do you see anything?"

"No."

"I am sorry. What do you mean? I am asking if you see any clots."

"It is up to the doctor. I just do the machine."

"You mean you can't tell?"

"I don't know, Ma'am. I told you already."

"When is this doctor going to look at it?"

"They will call you."

I found myself suspicious about her way of making the ultrasound films. I fantasized that she could do something to them, hide them somewhere, or swap them with somebody else's. I could not stop thinking about it in a sudden rash of paranoia. There are a lot of Jewish families from Ukraine and Moldova in the Philadelphia area. They are usually working class, unlike Jews like myself from Moscow and Saint Petersburg, who tend to be highly educated. Her parents were probably proud that she became a nurse. She was probably just a normal, Americanized immigrant girl from Russia, just doing her job. However, if she had wanted to sabotage my scans as a way to soothe any jealousy, any sense of the unfairness of life, I was certainly very vulnerable.

↭ III ↭

Nobody ever called me about the result. More days passed. Eventually, I called Dr. Blavatkez. He told me there were no clots and did not suggest any further tests or treatment. It looked like he was just going to leave me to suffer! My legs were in pain and I was miserable. It was very cold outside and I was constantly shivering, always in search of a warm place. After the phone call, I attempted to soothe myself by going to a bikram yoga place in town where the temperature was always kept very high. It felt good and warm, but I started to cry and cried through the whole class.

It had been years since the last time I'd cried. I felt safe. No one could tell there were tears on my face because it was so hot and everyone was so sweaty. I let tears fall for all the things that were wrong in my life: my horrible boss, my faulty rotting marriage, the unending pain in my swollen legs.

When, after my stroke, the doctors told me that it had been caused by clots in my legs I almost could not believe it.

CHAPTER 3
Speechlessness

In my room at the hospital, I was starting to feel much better. I had grown very comfortable with my inability to speak. Every doctor and nurse who attended me at Hope Memorial assured me that my speech would come back soon after I met with the speech therapist. I really was not worried at all. I was kind of excited because I saw it as a chance to get rid of my Russian accent.

Everything was fine, hilarious! Some multi-dimensional thread connected all things, and all things were the same. Nobody had to bother with sounds because there was no reason to divide the one, perfect, whole world. Trying to speak was like trying to paint without the concept of differentiated color, or to analyze a song playing on the radio without knowing the concepts of keys or notes. Why bother? It was freeing to just bask in the wonderful stream of ever changing all. For a little while, I was blissfully happy.

That day, they brought in the speech therapist, Dr. Heberholz. She looked at me and asked, "What is your name?" Gosha was in the room with me. "She can't talk," he said, "You know that, right?"

"She needs to talk, not try. Come on, tell me your name."

I think I must have waved Gosha out of the room and managed to make the first sound. I remember pushing sound through the debris in my brain and my mouth. Some kind

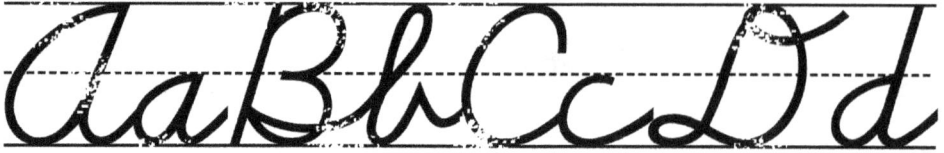

of uniting mush, disorganized trash, filled my head from
the inside. I could not tell where the mouth was or where
the brain was.

With a great mental effort I forced myself to get out of the
comfort of the mental snow and realize that at least there
were syllables: "L" and "A" made up the all-inclusive word
"La," which I used to count. "Mama" was La-la and father
was la-la and home was la, and so on. I knew it was not how
I heard words before. Dr. Heberholz must have known that
a patient who lost speech must be pushed and shaken and
required to make progress because, otherwise, they would
sink into the comfort of their own world of "la-la."

When my son wrote his name for the first time we kept this
piece of paper. His hand was unsure and shaky, but he was
proud. He brought it home from his Montessori School,
where they make children read at the age of 2 and do all
kinds of small things with their hands to develop their
brains. Looking at this writing I imagined him making this
effort, his hands not coordinated in doing what he wanted
them to, so I could imagine he was doing it very slowly,
letter by letter, sound by sound. I am guessing just the "S"
took him at least 5-10 minutes. The "I" perhaps 5. Then "M"
– must have been the most difficult one – the "M". Then
"O" came out almost perfect and round, and then "N" – also

Ee Ff Gg Hh

La

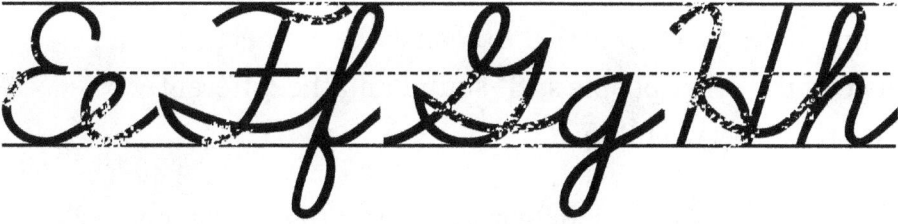

must be a difficult one—he must have spent another 5 or 10 minutes carefully directing the pen by his unwilling hand to do it. But then he did it and brought it home and we put it on the wall, where it is today. "So helpful!" I said, and I wrote with the same wobbly handwriting 'SIMON.' Because I started to collect sounds from LA-LA's into the shape other people meant for the sounds and letters to have – I started to collect the sounds for "SIMON" from that Montessori School. The timing and the labor of his writing it and me pronouncing and writing it were similar. The letters and sounds had to be pushed out carefully and with consideration, we both had to think about something that later would become a habit of a trained mind and body, but that was the moment of training, and it had to be very slow.

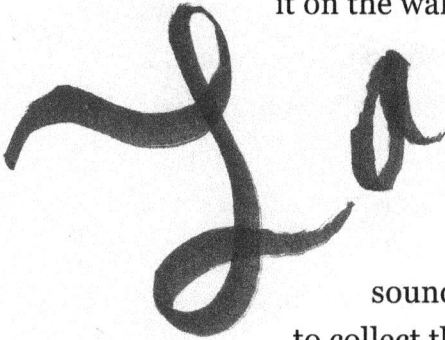

I had a picture in my mind of an S, in red marker, starting the row of letters to make up 'SIMON', all at the same height, and I pushed it out, "SSS" and an "I" next to it, and I thought about it and imagined the "I" and pushed it next to "SSS": "SS-III-"; I remember how the "M" was drawn, and I pushed the "M" out and the rest was easy "O" then "N": "O-N". S-I-M-O-N. I knew that I knew how to pronounce

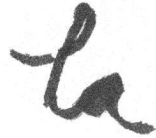

La

Simon's name, I knew it was not a bunch of "la-la's", so I think that was when I tried to realize the connection between the other people's "S" sound and the different letter that they meant by it.

Re-learning is harder than learning. After the stroke, my brain's connection to the comfortable abyss became strong as when I was a child and wanted only to play, resisting any work and any effort. After years of schooling, I became used to the ease of language and math, yet my brain could not grasp it. I remembered when it had been effortless and thought of myself as still being able to do it. Why would I have to try? My rational mind resisted the idea that I had changed. After the stroke, for whatever reason, the old ways did not work. However, the good news is that the brain is extremely adaptable, and it can re-route signals. New neurons grow and adapt. The main difficulty was to crawl out of the land of peace, an effort that felt so counter-intuitive, so problematic and unnecessary.

Dr. Heberholz left several pages of material I was supposed to finish by the next day. Strangely, it was not just my speech, it was also writing. I still, after three and a half years, struggle to write the way I used to, especially when it comes to numbers. This "la-la" for everything is still in my head, and sometimes it tells me that it does not matter which number I write because I understand that they are only symbols. I am still so tempted by the comfort of not knowing. That warm place whispers, "Never mind."

I encouraged myself with self-analysis and read books about language. What was I suddenly missing that I was unable to talk? I could still read. What was it I could not do, exactly, since I could read? Speech was a different thing altogether from understanding concepts, different from knowing words. I could see the walls built by others but I could no longer build my own. I had forgotten how to make bricks.

I spent most of my time completing the exercises the speech therapist left. They consisted of letters put together, then syllables. S-o, d-a-d, s-o-n, a-go, p-u-r-e. I did stacks of exercises and would see Dr. Heberholz every day for about a half an hour or so. My ability to speak slowly came back but, much to my dismay, so did my accent!

As I began to recover, in all ways, I started to crave exercise and would walk around with the line dripping heparin in my vein. The nurses were not against me wandering, greeted me, and even chatted. The nature of the stroke was still unknown. They were running blood tests every day, trying to figure out why my coagulation was so high. It was only after I started to regain my basic ability to speak, and to get bored with the speech therapy assignments, that I began to get nervous about my home life and the fact that the endless blood tests still had not revealed the cause of my stroke.

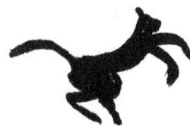

CHAPTER 4
Powerlessness

My sudden inability to speak seemed like a manifestation of my deepest frustrations. Gosha's mother moved in like a little Napoleon army, seizing the opportunity to take over my house. It finally was her house. As the new Queen, she requested, among other things, a microwave oven, "to feed the children." I hate microwave ovens.

"Honey," said Gosha one day, "I can't come because we are installing the new microwave oven."

"?"

"I already bought one."

I texted, "NOO."

"Don't worry, they liked it. Mom liked it."

Gosha's parent's liked grandiose, lavish things. Between this and Gosha's thriftiness I could imagine something awful.

"Ahh."

"It is beautiful and fits our kitchen and Mom likes it. It is silver and black."

I texted another, "NO."

"Honey, stop it. They said they needed the microwave. And,

I got it on sale."

"NO."

I hear him telling the folk in kitchen, "She doesn't like it."

"OK, got to run. Grandpa is waiting for me. Talk to Simon."

"NO! PLEASE DON'T!"

My son picked up the phone,"Hi Mom!
Don't be crazy. Dedushka is working hard.
We are laughing at you!"

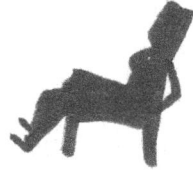

I heard them laughing.

"Mom, listen to this. Dedushka is drilling the wall. Do you hear?"

I heard something in the background. I heard their laughter.

Back then it felt so important to do things in my house my own way, to exist at least there, on the scene of my own household, not be dismissed in my own little kitchen land. I think I was too stuck up and fought for this little piece of dignity too much, but, alas, I did. I fought not to be dismissed. I was desperate and nobody heard me. In retrospect, not a victim, but a constant warrior fighting hard to be seen in her own battle.

⚜ III ⚜

Before I lost my speech, Gosha would often say when I felt there would a time for a discussion, "Honey, you are so inadequate that I will not even listen to you." Now, although he and his parents were genuinely sad for me, I could hear the little celebratory notes in their voices. Because finally this controlling woman lost her voice! I know they were sad for me, but they are also relieved to be the owners of my little land for a while.

The Queen was back, but she was an interim Queen. She did not know for how long though. Neither did I.

There was no point in debating.

When they installed the microwave, Dedushka, the master driller, stood on top of the new oven. Nobody noticed the surface was now bent. It was not designed for that kind of weight.

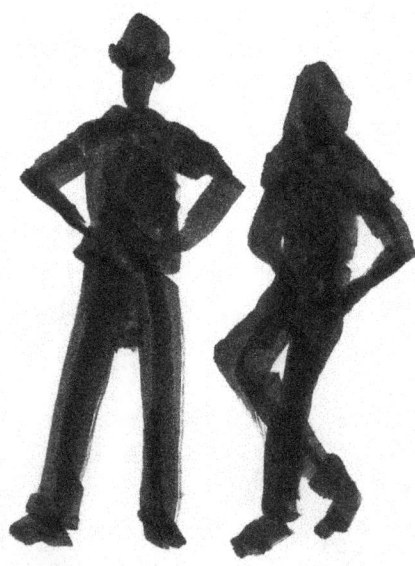

CHAPTER 5

My Children

At Hope Memorial Medical Center, there was a male nurse named Paul. This was the beginning of his nursing career. He laughed and joked all the time. He was so human, so refreshingly normal. He told me that he had just gotten married and that, since each of them had children from previous marriages, it was like growing a big family overnight. When I had my stroke, our neighborhood and school community and extended family came together to care for my children and they grew a big family overnight.

The word "stroke" was very scary. I tried not to think about it, but my children expected the worst. I could see it in their faces when they first visited me. Another mom, from Simon's class in Abington Friends School, had a stroke that put her in a wheelchair. My children were relieved and puzzled at the same time when I stood up from my hospital bed. They said nothing about it. They only carefully asked why it was I thought that I had a stroke. When I murmured something they said,"Aha."

The children were doing well. They were going to school and doing all kinds of normal things. I could tell, though, that they were waiting for something to happen and that they were scared. They looked silently horrified and silently hopeful. They were probably frozen by a sudden prospect of me disappearing, and perhaps played it out in their minds.

However, our entire network of acquaintances began

helping out, and my children suddenly found themselves surrounded by love and care. Neighbors and friends were bringing in tons of food. They were taking my children out to dinner, to concerts, to fun events. My dear friends organized summer camps for them: theater camp, circus camp. My friends did all the paper work, even applying for discounts. The circus camp awarded my children a free semester. The Breathing Room Foundation even bought my children school supplies.

My friend Lynn took the kids to see the landmarks of historic Germantown with her family. Her children and mine went to school together, and it was interesting to watch how children were handling the illness of a parent: these thirteen and ten year olds were compassionate and tenderly tactful. They were taught, early, the art of compassion and participation. My children learned this etiquette from being on the receiving side of kindness, but they know it now and exercise it when other people are in need. They do this with ease and grace. They can give too. They actually like it.

Love and kindness poured from everywhere around us. In the middle of a grave fear of losing their mother, my children knew that people were kind and giving. I am so grateful to all my friends, acquaintances and even strangers who came to our aid. My children will never forget this love, and they are eager to give back when they hear that somebody is in need. They learned love from the world.

In the life before I got sick, when I was a tortured soul, a friend recommended *Autobiography of a Yogi* by Yogananda, a famous book about the afterlife and reincarnation. I started reading it and played with its idea of being transported to a different place and a different life. I thought a lot about yogis and their practice of kindness. I thought about connecting to the mystical spheres that they believed existed. I asked Gosha to bring this book to me in the hospital and spent my days reading and meditating, cross-legged. At first, nurses were puzzled, but they quickly got used to me sitting on the floor and would not disturb me. Obviously it was better than me buzzing them all the time. However, as I finished reading the book, now in the hospital, I realized I chose this life and that I wanted the chance to live it. I wanted to be myself, in the place on Earth that I had made. And, more than anything, I wanted to be with my children.

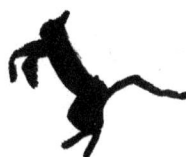

CHAPTER 6
No Diagnosis

Eventually, the hospital world sucked me into its well-oiled machine of processing the ill, into its smoothly operating belts and timely rotating wheels. I became part of the order within the walls. I would give my blood whenever I was asked. I would stretch my hand for the blood pressure muff. I would lie in bed, silent and surprised, no questions asked.

I

The room was nice. It had a separate bathroom, which I liked in spite of all the hospital rails and cord guards. The window overlooked the roof of a police station, a street, the roofs and lawns of small family homes all built in the 50's: all covered with a thin layer of snow. It was a cold February that year. I was hooked to a bag of saline and heparin on a rolling stand that I dragged alongside with me at all times: to the bathroom, to the window, to the hallway.

But, at the same time, I was an annoying, subhuman stick in the mud. Nobody could understand what was going on with me. I was trying to be a good patient, humbly waiting for somebody's authoritative decision, giving blood every day. The doctors at the heads of the morning processions took charge only to disappear in a day or two without giving me a diagnosis. I listened to them and answered their questions as best I could, but felt perversely responsible for being such a stubborn medical enigma. I was also becoming boorish and impatient. I became an Un-patient.

Gosha, without warning, became a caring spouse. He called the hospital several times every day. A friend of his, Tolik, a doctor, was actively involved. They spoke for hours each day about the particulars of my many blood tests. Gosha's boss, although he eventually chose to let Gosha go, visited me and organized food delivered to my house for the children while I was in the hospital. It was a bit uncomfortable to be exposed like that, but since I could not talk, I had no say. Everybody was frightened: transfixed by the possibility that something like this could happen to them, something inexplicable, undiagnosable.

I spent my days looking out of the window, reading, walking and waiting—as if it were a trial!—for the verdict.

At first, I waited silently, relying on the process and specifically refraining from interfering with it. Then I realized that something was not right with all these doctors' aloof proud silence. I started to ask questions. I even argued. Even though I could now speak, my words did not matter. I was ignored. It was only after I came to expect the quick exits from my room that I started to followed the doctors into the hallway with my questions, ready to catch a moment when the routine would be broken even for a second. "Sooo... Doctor Such-and-such... What is this new blood test telling you?"

The doctors looked very unapproachable. I could feel how the doctors felt important and how my questions damaged their surfaces. Successful doctors hard at work became speechless. I was avoided as much as anyone could afford.

It's the nature of things at a hospital. I was an extra, immobile, a gear in their clockwork. Or maybe I was more like an animal, alive, inside..."Doctor!"

"Yes..." The Powerful Holder of Knowledge would realize his slip, turn away, and nod to a nurse. She would yell at me, "Patient Gutkina! Go to your room!" I would argue with the nurse after I regained my speech.

"NO," I would say,"I am just trying to find out the result of my blood test."

"Patient Gutkina, you are not supposed to be in the hallway. Go to your room, or else."

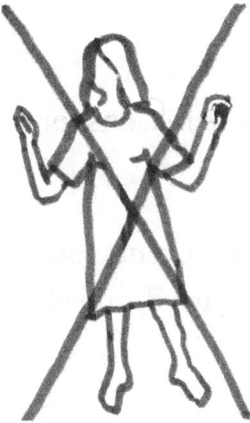

When I'd had all the nerve wracking I could take for the morning, I'd retreat to my room for breakfast. The people who brought the meals were always nice and talkative. They looked me in the eye and asked all kinds of questions. They were happy to rearrange my food on the tray as many times as needed, or to consult about the choices, or to help with napkins and silverware, or bring an apple, or stop by later to collect the dishes. Some nurses were nice, too. Especially later, when they realized that my hall wandering was harmless and that I was upset just as much as everybody else. They were always so overworked that I still do not understand how they managed to do all that they did: all those room calls, administering all those drugs, being of service in all other ways, and still returning each day to do it all over again.

᥍ II ᥐ

Although I was deemed a difficult patient, always asking questions, never in her room, I was not making progress towards finding out why I had had a stroke. Dr. Snyder talked about the mystery of the situation with me in the following terms:

"You know, people die all the time from unknown reasons."

I could not believe what I had just heard.

"Are you suggesting that the reason for my stroke will never be known? Or that I may die without even a diagnosis?"

"Very possible, very possible."

I didn't know what to say, so strange it all seemed. A professional, a doctor, content to not know the reasons for people's deaths?

"Also," he went on, "in many families, perhaps in yours too… Haven't you ever had an aunt or an uncle who just dropped dead? This is what I am talking about, Ms. Gutkina."

I was stunned. I considered this perspective. At that time, I did not reject any perspective or information of any kind. I absorbed everything that was happening around me, sometimes in awe, sometime in anger, sometimes with gratitude towards those people who were human in spite of the many opportunities the system provided to avoid feeling.

I was also examined by an American gynecologist, Dr. Barbara Patterns. She was very quick and very businesslike.

She immediately did an ultrasound exam, said that there was a cyst that might be just a regular menstrual cycle cyst, and concluded that she did not see anything abnormal. I must admit, I had not been having regular gynecological exams, but at this point that didn't even seem relevant. Barbara and I chatted about the gynecological office I used that went out of business recently. I recalled how one of the doctors there called me "Babe," and how she saved my daughter, during delivery, from suffocation by the umbilical cord. "There were issues," Barbara said, "but the doctors are still around." Chatting with this warm, personable doctor was calming and gratifying; she was professional, and she knew her field. She did not know I had cancer, and nothing she saw indicated anything was wrong. Had she known, for example, that I am the carrier of the genetic mutation that puts women at high risk of ovarian cancer, she would have done her exams differently. But no one knew that, yet.

This is a 45-year-old Russian female with no significant past medical history. She came into the hospital with not feeling well for the last 7 to 10 days. She complained of having intermittent chills, but no recorded fever, felt nauseous, experienced of vomiting and abdominal bloating, but no diarrhea. A day before of admission, she visited to the ER, but was sent back home on Levaquin for possible pneumonia. While in the ER, on the day of admission, she had started having difficulty finding words, was after being sent back home from the ER. Early in the morning, the next day, she could not type on her computer. She was having again the difficulty finding words. She called her husband who was at work. Husband felt she sounded confused as she told him she was dropping things from both of her hands. She could not dress herself. On the day of admission, the patient mentioned having still difficulty finding words. She denied any headache, any limb weakness, or any visual disturbance. The patient was normally fluent in English, but was not cooperative with history taking at the time of admission, saying she had already spoken to 6 people.

DISCEARGE SUMMARY

Now I am going to ask this: Why *didn't* anyone know that? Knowledge about the BRCA mutation was around for many years. It has been determined that women of Ashkenazi Jewish heritage are at high risk of carrying this mutation. The test had been available for a long time. Why wouldn't my primary care physician or my gynecologist suggest doing this test for me? I could have done something to prevent the cancer, or at least to have diagnosed it sooner. At this point, however, I was still in the dark about the fact that I actually had stage three peritoneal cancer. I was trying to wrap my head around the reasons for a stroke.

Gosha's theory, as he started to discuss with his friends, was that my stroke was a result of my laziness. When I left my job, he speculated, I slept too much and got stagnation in my blood. He neglected to consider that I jogged regularly all winter, but I felt so guilty for leaving my job, and then for getting so dramatically sick, that I even imagined he might be right. Guilt clouded my whole spectrum of feelings and thoughts.

**DEDICATION &
CERTIFICATION OF
THANKS TO:**

*Lynore, William,
Grant, Liam &
Siena Soffer*

**ANNA THANKS YOU FOR
YOUR KIND SUPPORT!**

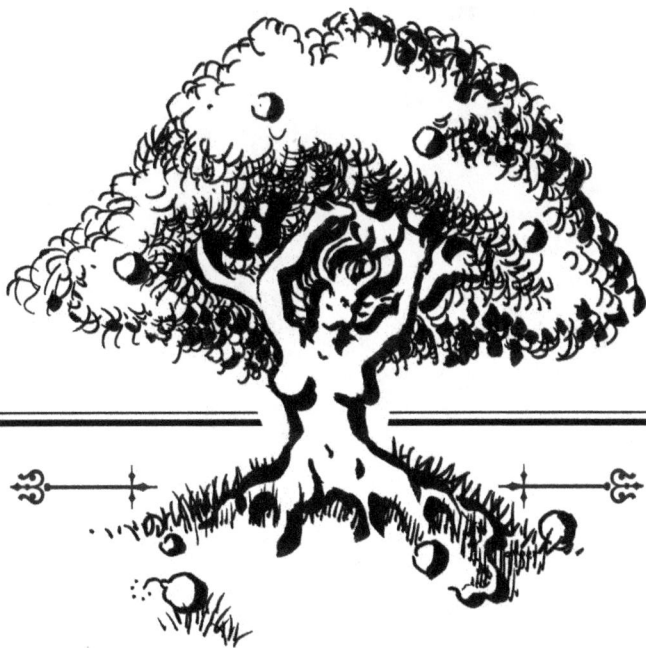

Doctors and Doctors

It was through a little hole in my heart that clots from my legs had traveled to my head and blocked the flow through certain blood vessels in my brain. Now it was official that I had had a stroke. Foramen ovale is a condition where the opening between chambers is not completely closed.

⟨ I ⟩

Doctor Slow, the neurologist who saved me with heparin, had intuited this diagnosis. He was somehow not on what they called my "team" anymore but, before he disappeared, he had ordered a heart exam. My team would come and go, day after day, pass by, check in on me, happy in their own Doctors' Lives, and distant in their expression of aloofness: the mark of their profession. They seemed to have no connection to the suffering they supposedly attended. They seemed proud of their achievements, their medical degrees. It seemed that nothing could shake their towers of self-satisfaction.

A Dr. Verma, who wore the demeanor of a general doctor in charge, seemed a little bit more involved at the beginning of our interaction than the others. She started by observing my nails and shaking her head as if in disbelief.

"What?" I asked her, really concerned and ashamed."

"Chipped," she said. "You see these white marks on your

nails? That's bad."

I thought she was kind and I hoped she could solve the mystery of my stroke. She told me she would be in charge of the team, gave me her business card, and left. I don't think I ever saw her again. That was usually how it went.

Then one day a hematologist was brought into my room. She immediately declared that she was married (to a medical doctor who practiced colonoscopy), that she liked to ski, and in fact was going on a trip really soon.

"Really?" said I. "Where do you ski?"

"I usually ski in Vermont."

"Oh, love Vermont," I said.

"Oh," she said. "How often do you go?"

"Every year, more or less. I like Canada too."

"Yeah. Mont Saint Anne. Love it."

"Love it too.

"But this time I am going to Colorado."

"Oh," I said.

She looked really well dressed; her shoes were the first thing I noticed when she walked into the room. A type of prep-school, JCrew girl – tasteful and expensively modest We chatted a bit about my illness and she said,

"No problem, we will order some tests that will help us. Don't worry. Come see me in two weeks."

"Two weeks?"

"Yeah. That's if you make an appointment today."

She was so girlish and vulnerable, that asking her about the gruesome details of the future tests seemed absolutely inappropriate, almost too invasive for her privacy. She left in a cloud of privileged assurance, a schoolgirl protected by her powerful Daddy or husband.

My team now included a neurologist (Dr. Brent Yoder DO), a gynecologist (Dr. Barbara Patterns), a hematologist (The Skiing Doctoressa Dr. Rebecca Prigoff), and an intern (Lagasse Sherman) and, last but not least—the remote invisible coordinator of the whole process—the family doctor from the office of Royal Dr. Weldon K. Moore (the Crying and Sad Dr. Louis Snyder).

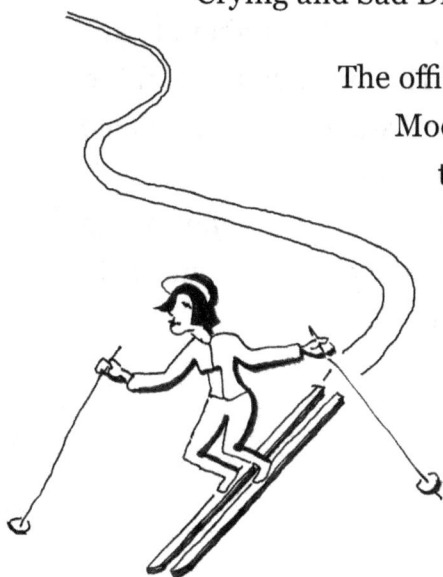

The office of Royal Dr. Weldon K. Moore sent Dr. Snyder after I said that under no circumstances would I see Blavatkez again. He missed the clots in my legs before I had my stroke and he was even looking for them! I could not bear to see him, at all. Just imagining taking his directions, and being subjected to his pseudo-thoughtful demeanor,

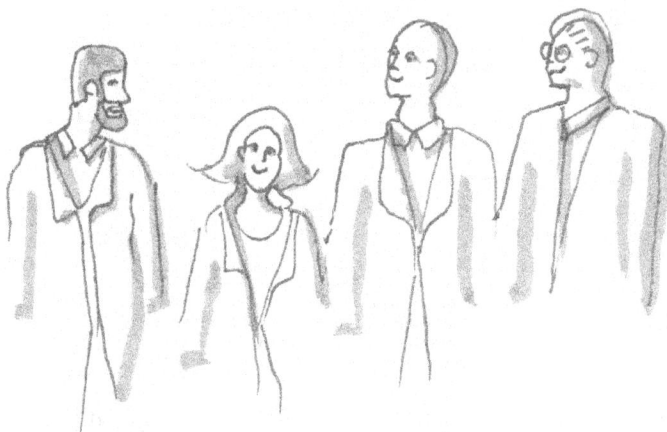

made me angry. I did not need yet another performance in which I had to participate and play the role of a patient! I did not feel like playing a role at all.

"I don't want to be seen by Dr. Blavatkes," I requested. Nobody objected. There might have been something in my voice that scared them.

But I would see Blavatkez one more time. He happened to pass by my hospital room on the day I was about to go home without a clear diagnosis. The only additional thing I could do was a CT scan a medical student had scheduled on a hunch. I asked him for advice. I don't know why. I'd promised to myself to ignore Blavatkez for his endless ignorance. I suppose I felt as if some fateful thread connected me to this trembling, fearful man.

✲ II ✲

Once upon a time, when I was getting ready to check out from the hospital, and was making farewell rounds in the nurses' hallway, saying warm goodbyes, providence sent a medical student from Temple University my way. If I recall correctly, he might not even have been part of my team. He might have been volunteering. One day, he appeared in my room and started to ask me the same million questions that I had already answered a million times. He had a couple of questionnaire pages with him. He sat at my bed side, which I never enjoyed. To me, it meant being a victim, and I avoided it whenever I could.

He continued to sit on my bedside,"Your name and date of birth? Do you smoke? If yes, how many cigarettes a day? Do you drink alcohol? If yes, how many times a day? Do you exercise? If yes, how many time a week? Are your parents alive? Do you have siblings? If yes, are they alive?" The third year medical student was nice and so polite. He told me the questionnaire was just for him, for his course study, and that he was really interested. I warmed up and decided to help him. He did not talk much, he just asked questions, and he was unusually polite and humble.

It was at this point that I was given permission to leave the hospital. I was ecstatic. My speech had mostly returned after a week or so of speech therapy, and there was no reason to think I was in danger of another stroke. I would continue to see Dr. Heberholz at her offices and was already scheduling visits.

I called the office of the hematologist, Dr. Rebecca Prigoff. An extremely rude receptionist told me that the closest appointment would be in two weeks. TWO WEEKS?! Again?! That was not an option, I thought. I tried, in vain, to negotiate for a sooner appointment. The receptionist was so rude, she actually hung up on me. I considered showing up at this office just to see the rude receptionist. I wondered what such a mean person could look like, imagining an unhappy woman: overweight, constantly snacking on something, and leaving crumbs on her bosoms.

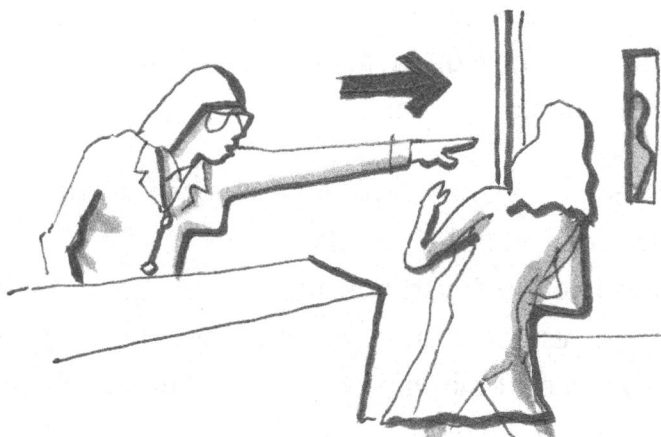

It was in this type of mood that the medical student found me on the day he stopped by my room and suggested a CT scan. "You know," he said, "coagulation can dramatically change with cancer. I am not saying that you have cancer. I'm just saying we should eliminate all the unknowns." I was preparing to be picked up, to go home at any moment. I was very eager to get started on my recovery.

This was when I ran into Blavatskez. He was so humble and so polite that I could barely hear his answer to my question.

"Yes, Ms. Gutkina, I think you should do the biopsy," he whispered.

I don't know why I listened to him, having discarded him as a medical authority, but I did. Although I hope he is no longer practicing medicine, and do not refer to him as a doctor for this reason, his good advice and regret at having failed me so egregiously redeemed Blavatskez, in my judgment.

As for the medical student, I have wanted to thank this young man for some time. His vision and timely advice were extremely important. Though just a third year student, he made the right analysis, the right decision, and he acted correctly. I wish I could meet him and thank him one day. Wherever you are, please continue to be smart, loving and human as you were when you helped save my life!

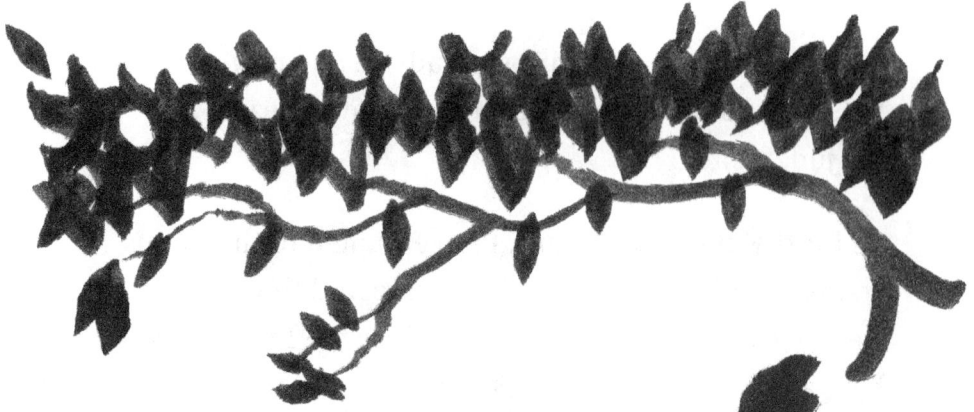

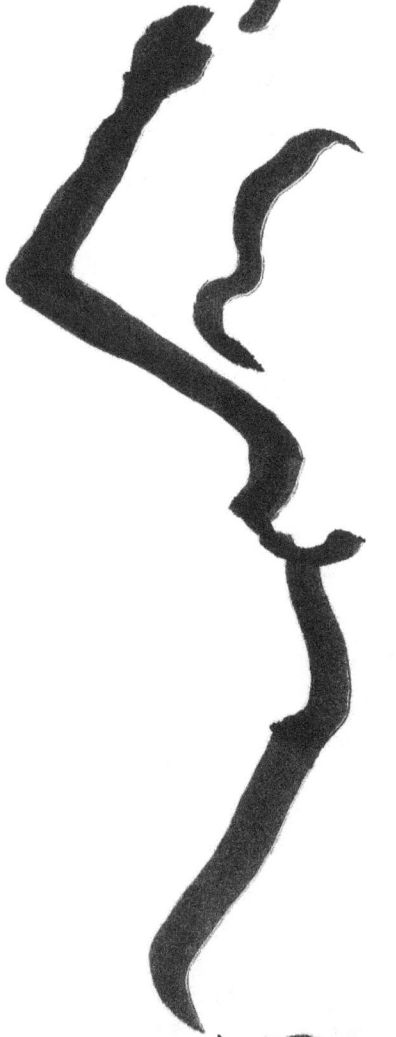

PART II

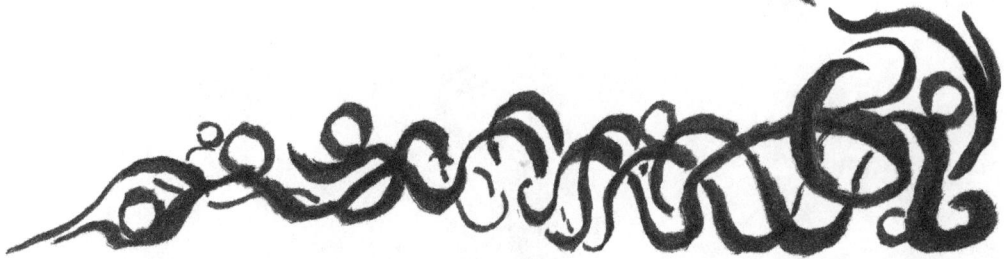

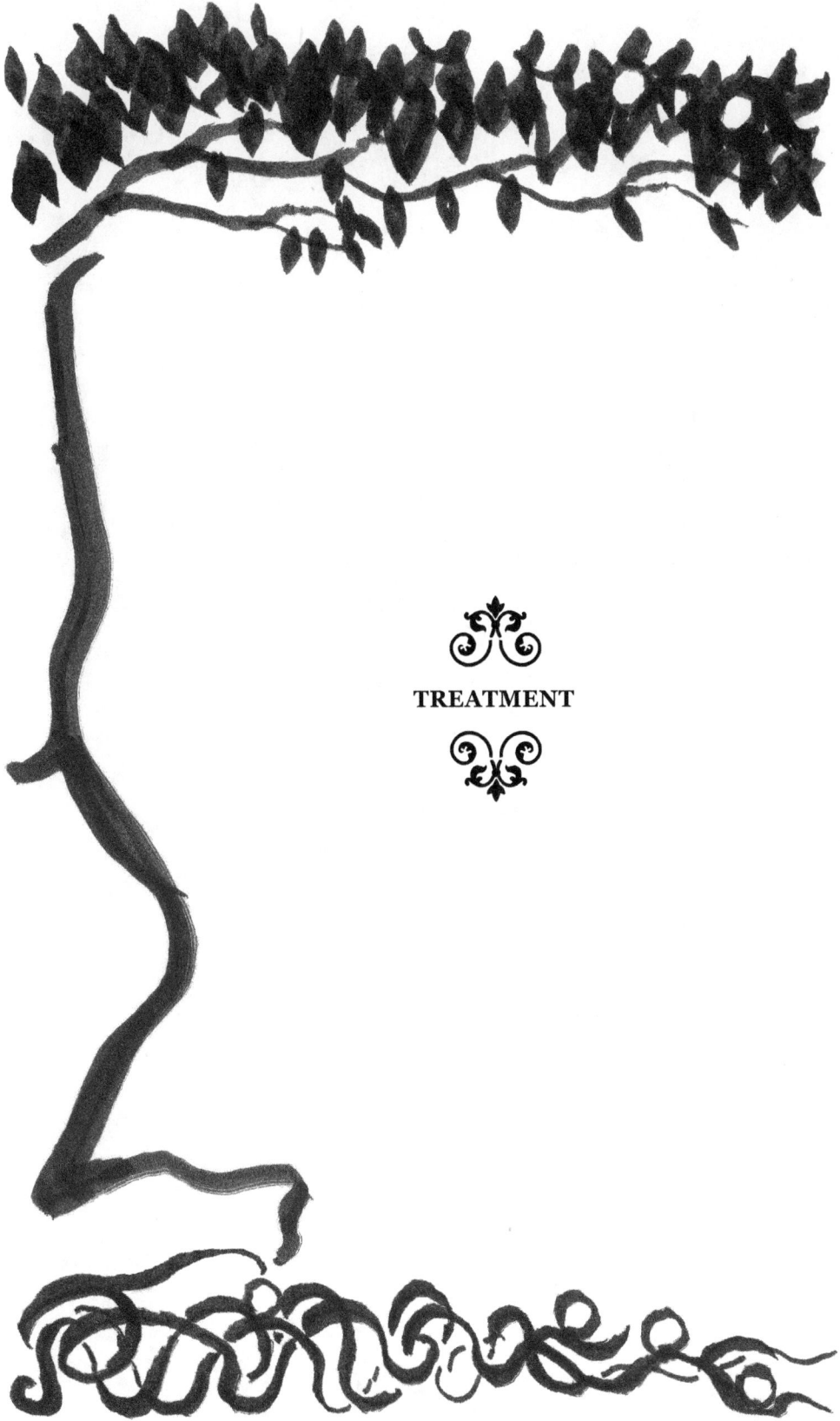

TREATMENT

CHAPTER 8

Stage Three

When I walked into Dr. Snyder's office, he hugged me and said, "I am so sorry. Anna, I am so sorry. You have cancer." He started to cry on my shoulder. It was quite awful. His job was to cure me, not cry on me! When I asked about the test.

"What kind of cancer?"

He kept on crying.

"I don't know."

"What do you mean you don't know?"

"Well, we just know from the pathology lab that the cells are malignant."

"What?"

"The cells are malignant and they are..wait...let me see... POORLY IDENTIFIED CARCINOMA."

"And?"

"It is very. Very. Bad."

He sobbed.

"But who would know?"

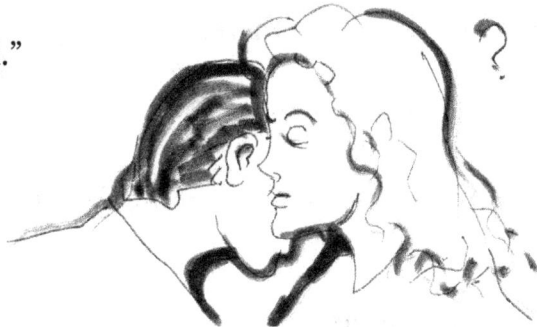

"Perhaps your hematologist, Anna. I don't know."

He handed me the pathology report, basically resigned to my imminent death.

Among the signs of malignancy scribbled on this lab test report was the fact that my cancer was stage three. That was when the race really started.

I broke the news to Gosha. He was devastated. I was afraid to tell this horrible news to the rest of my family. But he did it for me. Everyone froze.

I still had the appointment with the Skiing Doctoressa, who was working on my coagulation problem. Now she needed to take this new information and hopefully give me some idea of what kind of cancer I was dealing with.I called to make another appointment.

"Two weeks."

"Wait. I HAVE CANCER."

"TWO WEEKS."

"OK," I succumbed.

In two weeks I was there.

"How is the previous test?

"Nothing definitive," the Skiing Doctoressa said. "Let's do another one."

"In two weeks?"

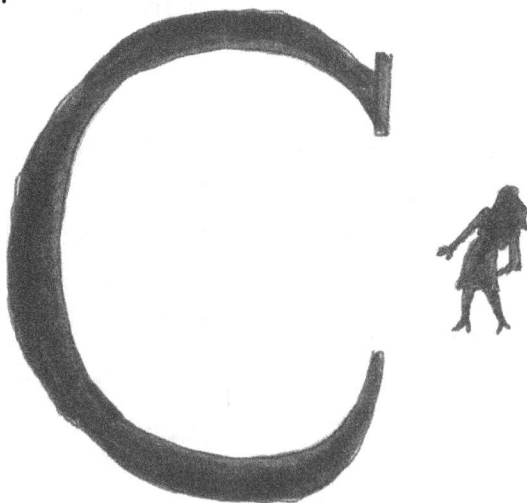

"In two weeks." Dr. Rebecca was going on a ski trip again. "Smiles."

I started to share the news of an unknown cancer with my closest friends.

My friend Connie heard good stories about a gynecologist at our local Hope Memorial Hospital. It was a random choice; He treated her friend of gynecologic cancer. It was the first oncologist that came out on the radar. By chance.

This time I did not call in to make a appointment. I asked my brother, an MD himself. The trick worked, and I got to see the doctor the next day.

Yahoo! That was something to start with.

The Recommended Local Gynecologist Number One was smart, and ordered five different tests at once. One test for each type of cancer. Results came back in a couple of days.

"CA125," he said at the appointment.

"What?"

"It means ovarian cancer."

"And what does it mean?"

The Recommended Gynecologist Number One was almost joyful as he told me what my future was going to be. First, I would undergo a round of chemotherapy that would work for a while. Then, I would have a recurrence and try a second round of chemotherapy. I would have yet another recurrence, really soon, and try a third round of chemotherapy, which would most likely not work. It would be completely my choice whether I would want to do the third round or not, but most people didn't. And, then what? I think I did not even ask, but it was obvious that this would be the expected and well-orchestrated end. I could not fathom that this was what I should expect. I left home devastated and immediately started to look for other doctors.

"Genetics is on my side," I thought. I came from a family of real survivors. After the battles of the Russian Revolution, purges of Stalin's elimination machine, World War II, another wave of purges, and many tricks and lures of the regimes, my family remained alive. And, they kept their humanity. I thought I had their ultimate strength, the iron innards of survivors.

My grandmother and my father, a five year old boy then, had stayed in the besieged city of Leningrad in the winter of 1941. There was nothing the authorities could do. People were dying from hunger. My grandmother's job was to count the heads of the survivors in the apartments on her street. She would take my father with her, always together—this was their rule—and they would do rounds. They would knock on doors and ask how many people were still living in the apartment. Then, my grandmother and my father were evacuated through the "Pathway of Life." A bunch of women and children were put into trucks. Crossing the lake, frozen over with ice, was the only route of escape from the besieged city. A truck ahead of them went under water, my

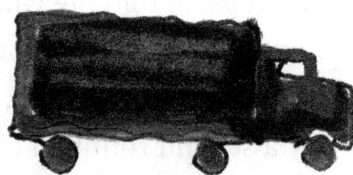

father told me, but their driver continued on. Separated from them, my grandfather survived the war and then eight years of Stalin's concentration camp. These were the kind of guts I expected myself to have.

Years ago, I read the book, *Cancer Ward* by Aleksandr Solzhenitsyn. It was a love story set in 1940's Soviet Russia, in Siberia, in Stalin's prison camp. I am very thankful to the author for the detailed account of his experience with cancer. He survived it, and lived a long productive life. His books provoked the fall of communism and the separation of Russia from other nations of the Soviet Union. But I adore books about love so, at the time, I skipped the chapters with cancer and read only the romance.

After my diagnosis, I ordered the book, again, and read the rest of it. Now, it was very useful, this attention to detail in a non-medical book. How long had my eyes been searching for this information in doctors' eyes, in waiting room brochures, in medical books? I loved that Solzhenitsyn described characters who did not have the desire to live, characters who were ashamed of their disease. His book offers a complete description, and is very useful as a guide through cancer's many faces, treatments, emotions, requirements for strength.

How alone Solzhenitsyn must have felt, back then. He broke silence and the stigma of cancer in the 1960's. I could not believe that, in 2009, my options were so unimproved! In the desolate hospitals of Siberia, the doctors were using the same techniques as now: radiation and

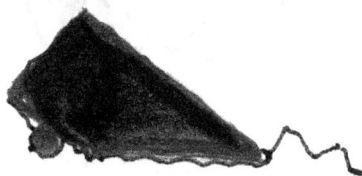

hormonal therapy. How is it possible, considering that thirty years of amazing technological advance has rapidly affected most aspects of human life, there has been no improvement in our treatment of cancer?

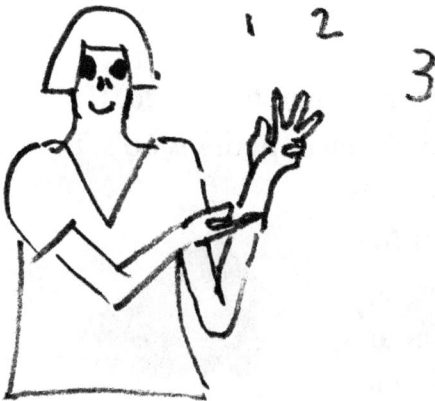

**DEDICATION &
CERTIFICATION OF
THANKS TO:**

Terry Jackson

**ANNA THANKS YOU FOR
YOUR KIND SUPPORT!**

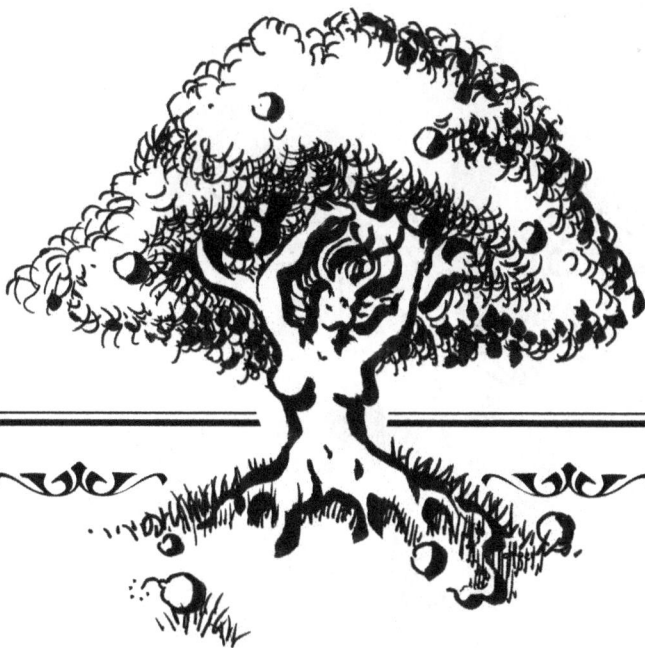

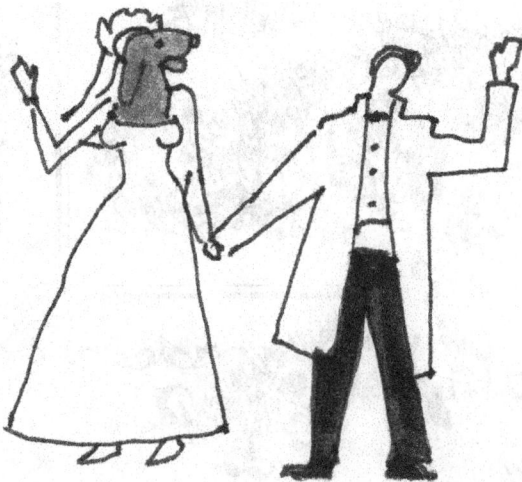

CHAPTER 9

Cheat

I suffered horribly the first time I sought a second opinion, which would be from a doctor I would travel to see in Baltimore. Warning: getting an opinion from a second doctor will feel like cheating on your lover. Looking back, I am proud of every second and third and fifty sixth opinion I got. The relationships between a patient and a doctor could be a lot like marriage – if you are afraid to break away. Or a lot like a dog-ownership – if you obey your master like a dog.

My first oncologist, the Recommended Gynecologist Number One had convinced me he was the only one who could help me. My appointment with the Baltimore Surgeon was eye-opening. This new doctor did not try to play me, did not stage his appearance in the room, did not roll his eyes, thunder his voice, whisper his insights, or employ any other tricks. Maybe it is not unlike the loyalty to your first lover: your first doctor. Unique, exceptional, cherished, he seems to be The Only One. The bond is hard to break and completely blind. A patient gazes at a doctor with loyalty that seems to have existed before they met. It is dog's love. Some doctors exude dominance, and some patients behave like smitten pleasers. I did. It is very easy to do.

Dasha, mother of a close friend, died in her late seventies. I think she died because she could not leave her first doctor, bound by this murky and fatal self-imposed loyalty. She resisted vehemently when her children begged her to get a second opinion from the best hospital in the area, the University of Pennsylvania. She waited and waited, scared of "cheating" on her arrogant and jealous doctor. He masterfully controlled her with love and anger—an American who spoke Russian to her! Then, it was too late to do anything. She died, on his orders, happily. When a patient refuses to get a second opinion, they risk their life. I know we all settle for all kinds of insufficient relationships in our lives. Most relationships are imperfect, complicated, sometimes abusive, mutually exhausting.

The good doctor at the hospital in Baltimore spoke plainly about my health and options. He was willing to be my doctor, but he was not hunting for patients. He said he could perform the surgery, but chemo... "Why bother coming here? It is all the same everywhere, anyway." It was my first honest encounter with the notion of standard treatment. I learned that any doctor at any hospital would prescribe the same chemotherapy drugs for ovarian cancer. "I am not a God," the best of doctors would say, and "Nobody can tell you how long you have to live," and "You are a strong person. You'll be ok." That last would be my favorite. I hated the scare tactics of my be first manipulative doctor and had no more time for him.

All partnerships are life and death collaborations. We should not be afraid to leave, if we want to be alive. Strangely, we resist our power: numbed by the slowness of events, paced by the absence of obvious alternatives. It is life that slips away, every day we succumb to struggles and animosity.

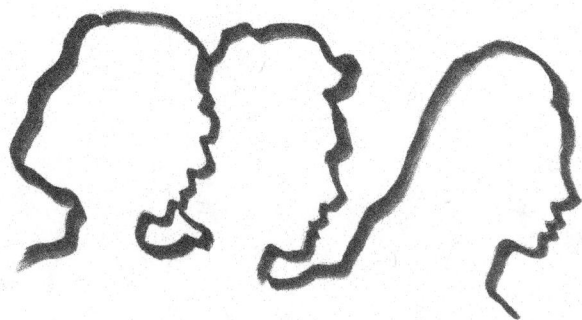

CHAPTER 10

Support

My family started to put in an enormous effort to help me. My brother bought my Mom a ticket, and she came from Russia. We assigned her the task of making a glass of carrot juice for me twice a day, which she did religiously. Someone had given me a video where a woman cured herself with carrot juice. She drank two to three glasses every day, and was fine in the end. So, I drank carrot juice. My mother was also indispensable in making meals for the children. This was the first time I let go. I let others check on my children's bed time, their homework, their music lessons. I was freed to focus on my research, appointments, the endless weighing of options. My father and uncle spent hours with me, talking on the phone. They shared my frustration, and that made it bearable.

I tried to hide the fact that I had lost my speech. I tried to hide the fact that I had been in the hospital for weeks. The people I tried to hide these facts from were my parents, my ninety-three year old grandmother in Russia, and my uncle's family in the US. It would be too embarrassing to be seen to be so weak, so unfortunate, such a failure. Also, I didn't want anyone to worry about me. I had already complained, too much, about my unhappiness that fall and winter. I had complained about my bullying boss, my stubborn husband and my loneliness. Adding an undiagnosable condition after a stroke? It would be too much for my conscience to burden them with.

I do describe all these events as a scientist. All the details may seem irrelevant to my dendritic vaccine, the primary subject of this story. But as a scientist I find it necessary to describe as many seemingly unrelated facts as possible so that the next thinker would take my accurate diary of events and find some new patterns and relate the seemingly unrelated facts in a new way, perhaps leading to a solution.

And the full picture of my cancer is that right before I got sick I did not get along with my father, my boss, and my husband. These "un-relationships" were like a wound that would not heal but would get worse with time.

Perhaps this bitterness had something to do the hormonal signaling that allowed the cancer. Perhaps bitterness weakens the immune system. I am sure in a couple of years we will know exactly what chain of hormones, cytokines, and other molecules causes this Ultimate Melancholy Condition.

That winter I was complaining to my family a lot.

Whenever in my life I had complained about the unhappiness brought on by my boyfriends or husbands, my mother was always supportive. She had been betrayed by the men in her life, too, and believed they were the reason for her unhappiness. At seventy five, she still carries the expression of a child who has been a unjustly punished. In her youth, she was stunningly beautiful and very smart. She was also very romantic but, in the end, she found herself alone. Life was different from what she thought it ought to be, as if the rules had changed in the middle of the game. She was always on my side, when I questioned my father—his style, his intentions, his integrity—just as she was on my side when I questioned the integrity of other men in my life, when I blamed my failures on them.

My grandmother, not surprisingly, took the side of tradition. She was not sympathetic to any of my marriage complaints. She was not sympathetic to any of my career complaints. No matter how detrimental to my well being, marriage was the thing to work on. In spite of my efforts to hide the fact of my hospitalization and my illness, the nature of which was unknown, the Russian part of my family found out about it. I imagine it was my mother-in-law who shared the grim information. So, the moment I was released from the hospital, she instructed me very strictly, "Stop whining, and get back to your family. Get back to your children."

My career had been effectively ended by a jealous, manipulative boss. Nothing had prepared me for that. I had never been ambitious until I started to really succeed. I had been like an observer, more interested in life and relationships. My corporate success surprised me. I liked it, but my boss disapproved. His tenuous suspicion, his jokes, his denial of the value of my ideas and my contribution: I complained about these to my father. He had always been an ambitious career warrior, always fighting for his ideas. Who else would I turn to for actionable advice? My mom's would not be relevant, since she never really pursued a professional career. Although she was very smart and quick, she was not ambitious.

Surprisingly, my father was rather cold when we talked about my troubles with my boss. There was a contrast between his frozenness on the subject of my career and warmth on the topic of my family. The latter would always excite him. "No. You better tell me about the kids. That's real," He would derail my career conversations. Soon, I stopped talking to him at all. I sensed him being "on the guys' side."

"Oh,"my mother would say when I shared the suspicion with her. "How can that be? He loves you so much." I did not know how it could be. It was a big puzzle for me. But, in this battle for my identity, my father was on the side of the status quo, the side of traditional gender roles, the side of other men. By the time I got sick, I held a huge grudge against his betrayal. I had already discovered that my husband's loyalties were the same as my father's. The truth was hurtful and sad. I complained and whined a lot.

My grandmother survived the Revolution, hunger, the war, the siege of Leningrad and never took pity on me. She did not even want to believe I had cancer. "Don't kill ME," she would say. "Don't say that. How can it be?"

My father, though, completely turned around. He was no longer watching my struggles from the sidelines. No longer aloof and intimidatingly indifferent. But cancer was a serious enemy, and we re-united. He became one of the major people in the army of people who helped me, day after day. So did Gosha. So did all the guys.

Taking sides is always a source of frustration. It was me that bitter winter – calculating who is on my side and seeing that nobody was. Except when the cancer struck. Then everyone was on my side.

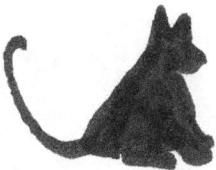

CHAPTER 11

Hospitals

In my search for the doctor who would become my primary physician, I vetted a great many hospitals. Sloan Kettering has a reputation for being one of the best hospitals in the country for cancer treatment. I sent them the scans, the biopsy report with the stage three indication. By then, if waiting for a hospital to get back to me, I'd start looking for another hospital to assess. I had had so much of my time wasted, been made to jump through so many hoops, and dealt with so many incompetent or otherwise problematic professionals, that I had learned to keep the standards for my selection of hospitals and doctors extremely high. I'd learned to require a certain feeling of being cared for.

When a hospital did get back to me, later, I would evaluate them on relevance and speed. I did all this intuitively, feeling it out. I think Sloan Kettering did call back but, since I did not go there, I assume it was not meaningful or helpful. So many hospital decisions are made by nurses and junior doctors who have never met you. You think they would work for you but actually they are working for a hospital, with its own complicated and challenging operations logistics. Obviously, they don't look out for your interests. They need to calculate on the spot whether your living body will add something valuable to their operations or will be a drag on their resources. Calculated on the spot and using the criteria that their operations dictate. When I was communicating with Sloan Kettering I felt that I bumped into the wall of an unknown formulaic regulation that did not let me get into the system easily. I gave it up after several rounds of sent documents and phone calls. I was still not good on the phone with numbers and dates, the remaining complications from the stroke, and they were clearly irritated by my slowness.

Maybe if I had found a doctor there whom I knew through a friend, it might have been a different story... But for an outsider like me—it was not worth my time.

The Gynecologist Number One sent me to do another scan – this time a PET scan. I remember the young doctor at the monitors, with attentive and sad eyes. Perhaps he was saddened by my diagnosis. Somehow, the scan showed no malignancies... "Hmm, "said Gynecologist Number One, "With ovarian cancer, it's tricky. It doesn't always show up on the PET scans."

He said he wanted to make sure I don't have any other cancers and sent me to his friend at the local office, one of those Local Hospital Associates types with long lines and a secretary so mythically angry you immediately start to kiss up to her and try to make her smile. The exam did not reveal anything wrong with my digestive system. But "just in case" they suggested that I should schedule the colonoscopy.

On my way out of the office, I met some friends. "What are THEY doing here?" I thought, and perhaps they thought the same about me.

I was bleeding profusely by then and was getting weaker by day.

All that time, I was on blood thinners. They suggested I should buy a fashionable emergency bracelet that would announce my being on blood thinners – to the paramedics. In case I am in a car accident. The bracelet had a scary aesthetic: Harley Davidson goes military. It was too strange and I did not buy it. On the drive to Baltimore to Gynecologist Number Two, with Gosha, I was agonizing about the absence of the bracelet on my wrist. What if we get into an accident... I would be bleeding... the paramedics would not know why... and then Gosha would say that we should not worry about that yet, and that we were likely to get there safely.

Gosha was a loyal companion, but he would usually cry in a doctor's office and this was one of the last times I took him with me. All the books and all my friends suggested that I have someone with me at the appointments, to help ask questions, for a second pair of ears, for a second judgment. Gosha was a perfect help, in many other respects, but horrible at the appointments. Doctors managed to intimidate him into complete submission very soon, with their tactics of patient intimidation. He would let me ask questions. Then, he would sit there and cry. He could never remember much of the conversation for later analysis, or take notes, or scrutinize the doctor's words, or ask questions that would help me make an informed decision.

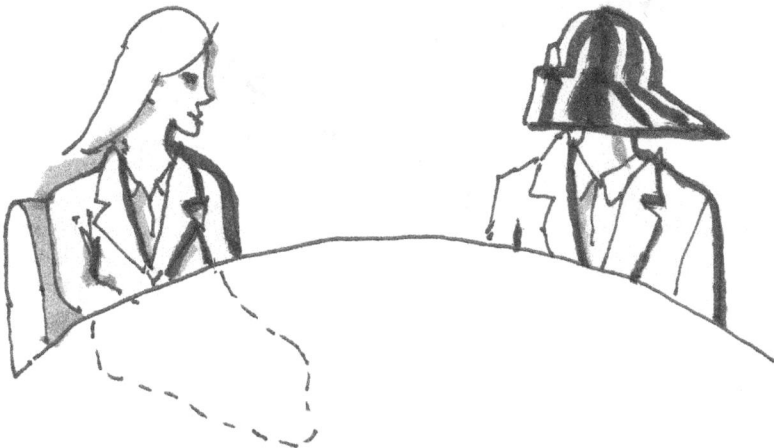

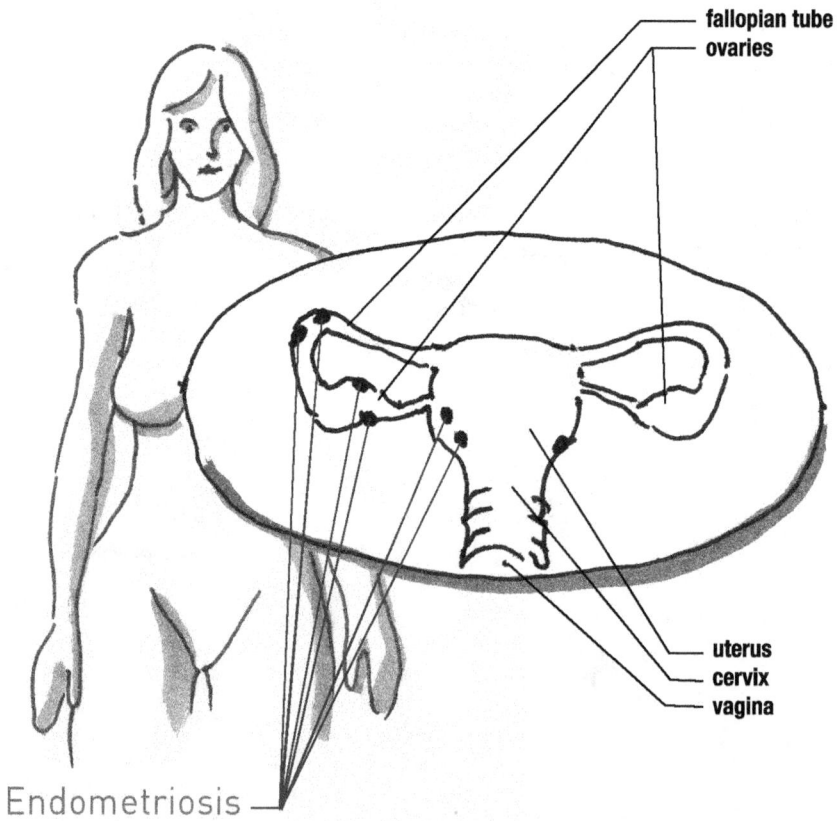

fallopian tube
ovaries

uterus
cervix
vagina

Endometriosis

CHAPTER 12

Association

Annette, a friend of mine, had cancer a year before me. I saw her at the store with her head shaved, and I did not say, "Hi." Later, she helped me find the right doctors, the right nutritionists, herbalists, etc. She actually handed me her contact list of reliable specialists. But, the first time I learned she was sick, I ran away.

The news that I had cancer changed my outlook on life immediately, and this outlook keeps changing. That night, I went to bed feeling about to die and I woke up in denial. It could not be happening to me because...it just should not. I suspect that feeling is common, among the newly diagnosed. The shock separated me from my life, completely, as if I was already dead. I remember I would go to the bathroom and moan in disbelief. When I was sleeping, I still remembered. It ran on the background of my dreams and, when I would open my eyes, the hard knowledge—"I have cancer"—would awaken me for a day of moans.

Of course, I knew that many other people before me had been in the same situation, and I had always been unsympathetic, arrogant. I had felt invincible. I had never donated to a cancer charity. In my Soviet Darwinian superiority, I would never have considered giving to those in need. I remember several occasions when co-workers were involved in cancer donations and, every time, I babbled some excuse, some intentionally transparent lie. I thought charity was a weird extortion, an American game.

I was not going to play at all. Now, I see that my stinginess was rooted in fear: the fear of touching anything related to cancer. I was afraid to be associated with it at all. Also, cancer taught me about giving. I relaxed my possessive fist.

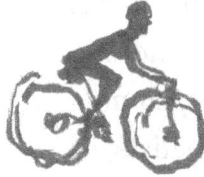

∼ I ∼

When my uncle found out about my cancer, he mailed me Lance Armstrong's book about his cancer journey, and it changed my attitude one hundred and eighty degrees. *Not About the Bike* includes all the details about Armstrong's life: his girlfriends, his mother, his stepfathers, friends, the story of his diagnosis, his multiple attempts to grasp what was happening, his realization that sometimes his doctors only pretended to know what to do, his long resistance, his surrender, his flight to another state to do chemotherapy, his weakness, the risks that he had to take to find his cure, his new life after cancer, his new career in charity, his new wife, her artificial insemination, and their baby. All of it was equally important. Equally important.

There would be fantastic similarities between Armstrong and myself, in how we weathered the journey, in how people helped, in what roles they played. This book told me to open up to friends, and to be tough in my search for the best doctors, for cures, for opportunities that friends bring in, for honesty with myself and the belief that there is light at the end of the long tunnel.

There was an episode when he was ridiculed for his lack of masculinity, as the result of removing a testicle. I would have a very similar episode myself, when a woman journalist would ask me about my cancer. I told her it was ovarian cancer.

The same thing happened, long after my surgery, when I shared the story of my cancer with a local woman journalist. She is so brilliant that I did not even feel I was being interviewed.

"What type of cancer?" she asked me.

"Ovarian."

"Wow, and what did they do? Did they take all that stuff out?"

"Yes," I said.

She immediately moved on, interviewing other people in the room. I am also Jewish, and I know how much the ability to give birth is emphasized in the Jewish tradition, and I almost understood her disgust at knowing this detail about me. But I think she missed an interesting story, having left so early!

This dialogue with the surgeon is still fresh in my mind.

"What are you going to cut? Please, I am begging you. If it is possible, don't take out everything."

"We'll see," Dr. Mayor replied.

"What do you mean, 'We'll see?' I want something left!"

"We'll see. Get ready. You will be okay."

And, of course, the cancer was spreading in the peritoneum, both ovaries, fallopian tubes, and even the kidneys. Dr. Mayor had to remove my core birth-giving organs.

❧ II ❧

In the new hospital, I felt like I was in good hands. I also had confidence in the anesthesiology team that had to monitor my heart closely to prevent rapid pressure change, which could cause possible clots to travel to a wrong chamber. My brother, who is an anesthesiologist, instructed me on what I had to ask from them. I think he might have spoken to the head anesthesiologist, himself, too.
Just in case, I told them what I understood. They listened very attentively, and took many precautions. They also inserted a filter for catching clots. When I returned to the hospital, some weeks or months later, the experience was in such wonderful contrast to my other hospital experiences that I considered it a pleasure!

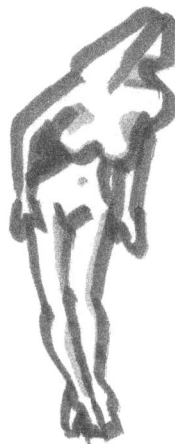

The idea of losing my reproductive organs horrified me. I did not know that my sense of self was so centered around my womanhood. If I had had time to think about it, I'm not sure I would have gone through with the surgery! I might have chosen to die! I felt that the part of me the surgeons were going to remove was the part most dearly myself. I felt lost. I didn't plan on having more children. I was forty seven years old and nearing menopause anyway. It had nothing to do with the future, and everything to do with my sense of identity.

I was hit especially hard because, right before I was hit by cancer, I had been focused on my own femininity and childbirth, and I studied the reproductive system in Gray's Anatomy. I wrote about it. I refreshed my memory of my college biology studies, of anatomy and of embryonic development. I found it very romantic and very essential to imagine my own embryonic development, the warmth of my mother's womb, and my journey through the birth canal and emerging into the world as me, self, a person. I played with this in my writing. Now the joke was played on me, on my ovarian fixation, as if fate was watching me with a dare. "Now, what are you gonna do?!" Like a demanding teacher.

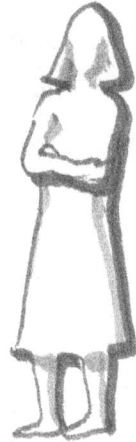

Serendipitously, I am writing this in my favorite spot in Jenkintown, the Jenkintown library, and the young woman at the table in front of me has a presentation open on the reproductive system. Looking over her shoulder, I can see the familiar symmetrical diagram: two ovaries, like two grape bunches, the fallopian tubes like vines joining into a central cup—the womb—and, beneath it all, the vagina, acting as both beginning and end to the loop. Now that I have time to look at this again, I see it from a different perspective. So many things can go wrong! How vulnerable all these different tissues are.

Fallopian tubes: Each tube is about 10cm long. The width varies at different parts along the length: thinnest at the ovarian end, more *muscular towards the uterus. Its widest part, the **ampulla**, is adjacent to the **fimbria**. The ampulla's importance lies in the fact that fertilization of the **ovum** by the sperm usually occurs in this region.*

The fallopian tubes are also the site where blockage most commonly occurs, leading to infertility.

***Ovaries:** The two ovaries are situated on either side of the **uterus**. They are the female sex gonads and are responsible for the release of a mature ovum every month (ovulation). They are also the chief producers of the female sex hormones: estrogen and progesterone.*

*The ovaries are pinkish-white in color and roughly oval in shape, being 3cm in length, 2cm in breadth and 1cm in thickness, approximately. Each ovary has a thick outer lining, called the **cortex**, and an inner part, called the **medulla**. During the reproductive life, i.e. from puberty to menopause, the cortex contains numerous **Graafian follicles** at different stages of development. Every month, a Graafian follicle in one of the ovaries matures and releases an ovum. This phenomenon is called 'ovulation.' During a woman's lifetime, only about 400 follicles reach maturity.*

Any of these cortexes, endometrial handles, ligaments or follicles can go wrong.

Before the surgery, before my cancer diagnosis, I enjoyed the mysterious power of being female. I felt it deeply, but had no conscious understanding of how much it meant to my sense of worth, to my sense of self. Years after my surgery, I am thinking about this for the first time. With the anatomical loss—loss of my ovaries—I transcended being a woman. I became a human being.

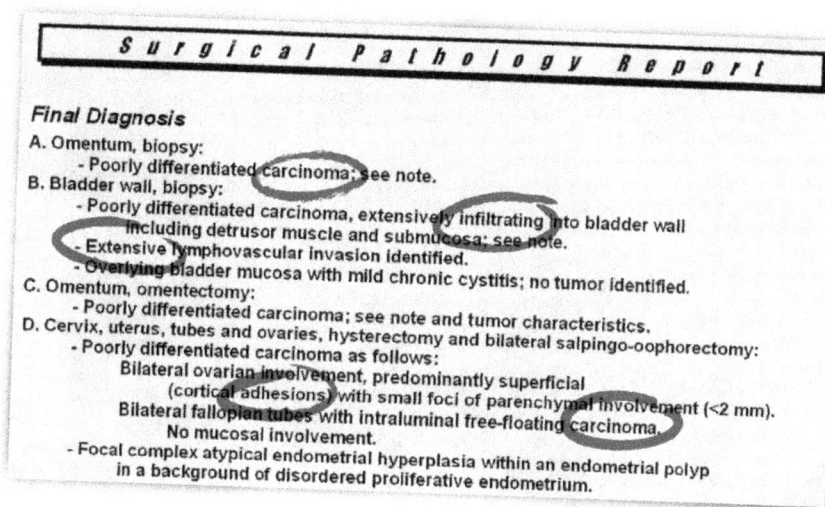

Surgical Pathology Report

Final Diagnosis

A. Omentum, biopsy:
 - Poorly differentiated carcinoma; see note.
B. Bladder wall, biopsy:
 - Poorly differentiated carcinoma, extensively infiltrating into bladder wall including detrusor muscle and submucosa; see note.
 - Extensive lymphovascular invasion identified.
 - Overlying bladder mucosa with mild chronic cystitis; no tumor identified.
C. Omentum, omentectomy:
 - Poorly differentiated carcinoma; see note and tumor characteristics.
D. Cervix, uterus, tubes and ovaries, hysterectomy and bilateral salpingo-oophorectomy:
 - Poorly differentiated carcinoma as follows:
  Bilateral ovarian involvement, predominantly superficial (cortical adhesions) with small foci of parenchymal involvement (<2 mm).
  Bilateral fallopian tubes with intraluminal free-floating carcinoma.
   No mucosal involvement.
 - Focal complex atypical endometrial hyperplasia within an endometrial polyp in a background of disordered proliferative endometrium.

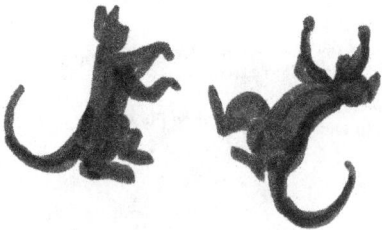

CHAPTER 13
Recovery

The surgery was over, and I was to spend some time in the hospital before I could go home. I woke up in my room and the pain kicked in. Then, it increased. Gosha was with me. He rushed to get the nurse. The nurse came, and I told her my pain was intolerable. I was yelling and squirming, in my bed, pressing the buzzer like crazy.

"What's wrong, Honey?" Gosha asked

"Oghhh!!! If you don't get the nurse, I will die. Oghhh!!! I will sue them! Tell them, I am suing!"

Gosha rushed to the nurse's station. After an insufferable interval, a nurse arrived.

"What's wrong, Ms. Gutkina?"

"If you don't get me the doctor, I will call the police!"

"Are you in pain Ms. Gutkina?" the nurse asked.

"Yes! Do something now! Please! Please!"

"You are already getting the maximum allowed amount. It is too late to call the doctor now. He is out already."

And the bitch left the room. Of course, she had other patients, but I bet she didn't do anything for any of them, either. Some nurses have no patients because they have so many.

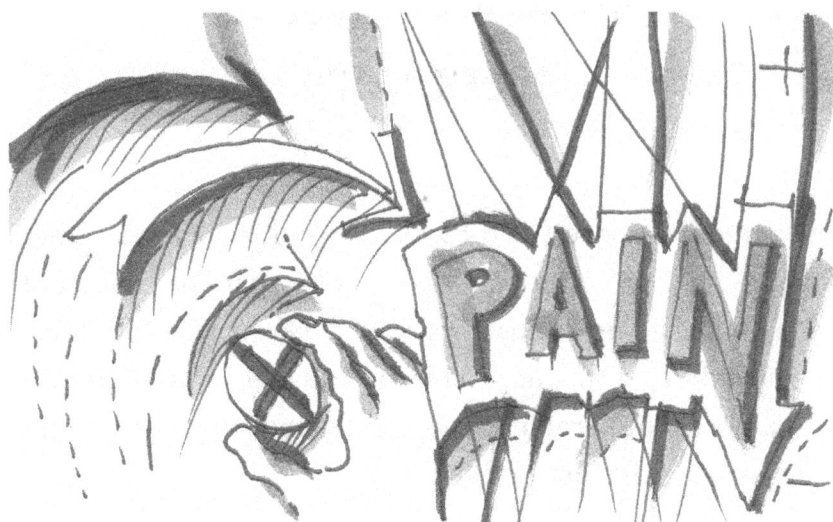

"Gosha, do something!" I screamed in unbearable pain.

"Ogh, Honey. Your pain threshold must be really low," he said.

I was turning the dial on the manual thing that they gave me to regulate morphine, but it did not help.

"What is going on?"

Gosha went to the nurses' station again. The same nurse returned.

"Ms. Gutkina, I already told you. The regulations are such that you can only increase the concentration of the pain killer once every 5 minutes."

"No, it's not possible! You can't have me here, dying!"

"You are not dying, Ms. Gutkina."

"I am telling you, I am!"

It was horrible. I screamed. Finally Gosha made her increase the amount, for a short period of time. It felt much better.

I stayed in this hospital for about a week, waiting for signs of improvement. My friend, Mark, brought friends to visit. They all took pictures with me, in the high hospital bed. I hope they did not see the line that attached my bladder to the collector bag. We made goofy faces for the pictures, and it felt really good to laugh.

Gradually, I was taken off the IV and started on oral pain killers. Because some surgery was done on my bladder, I was attached to a urine collector pouch. The pouch filled with urine by itself, but it was not visible. It fit on my leg, and was covered by my skirt. I was told it was a temporary thing and that it would be removed, soon. I think I had it for quite some time, maybe a month or so, but nobody noticed. One time, the stint fell off. I was in the middle of a meeting. I had to excuse myself to the bathroom and re-attach the tube.

The people with whom I was talking probably guessed what I was doing in the bathroom for so long, but it wasn't otherwise inconvenient. It is amazing how well developed the art of fixing people up is, and how ingenious all these seemingly horrible devices for hiding ugly bodily inconsistencies are. "Before" I would have cringed. But the humanity of the medical system brought to life so many devices that people don't need to lose their dignity over your bladder emptying into a bag. A simple and ingenious thing! But if not for this, I would have been bed ridden for months. It depends on how you look at it.

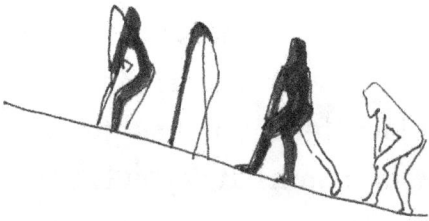

CHAPTER 14

Rest

After the surgery, I was sent home to rest and heal. It seemed like a strange proposition. On one hand, I was rushed to start chemotherapy on my rapidly spreading cancer by all the doctors I have seen; on the other, I was told to do nothing about the cancer for a month after the surgery. That made no sense to me. Why didn't they stop the cancer first, with chemotherapy, and then do their surgery? I kept posing this question to my surgeon. Instead of getting the answer, I got a reputation for being crazily tenacious. Besides, Dr. Mayor told me, his job was done and my next step would be chemotherapy with the oncologist. I was sent home, for a month, and not permitted to do anything but heal.

I remember lying in bed and looking out the window. It was March of 2009. The huge maple tree in my yard was bare and gray, shaking its branches in the wind. I had never really looked at this tree before. Now, I stared at it for hours on end. I guess I really didn't feel very good, because I didn't mind staying in bed. I would get up, take a shower, and then go back to bed. Eventually, I was encouraged to start walking. That was not easy. The surgery was so extreme that I needed to heal for a long time. Finally, I made it out on the street. I walked very slowly. I barely made a circle around my block. I never noticed, before, that one street was on a slope. I slowly climbed, painfully aware of how unusually hard it was. These fifty yards took me a long ten minutes. I could not breathe well. When I called the doctor with the update, he told me difficulty breathing was to be expected. I calmed down. I had been worried. I had never had difficulty breathing before.

My neighbors watched my walks, with awe. They were used to seeing me jogging. Even in November of the previous year, before I started to feel bad, I would run for about an hour. One woman came up to me and asked if I was okay. I could not speak, but started crying. She understood, and cried with me. Then she would stop by from time to time, to ask if I needed anything. I was so grateful for all the kindness that poured in. Gradually, I was walking again, even meeting people. Most of them did not have any idea that I had recently been in the hospital but quickly figured it out and always offered sympathy.

A pastor of a church on my street once stopped by on a tip from a parishioner. I was crying as we sat in our living room. I always succumb to a sympathetic listener.

In another local church my friends were praying for me with their congregations...

I was getting a real team around me.

**DEDICATION &
CERTIFICATION OF
THANKS TO:**

Maria &
Alexandra
Nilova

**ANNA THANKS YOU FOR
YOUR KIND SUPPORT!**

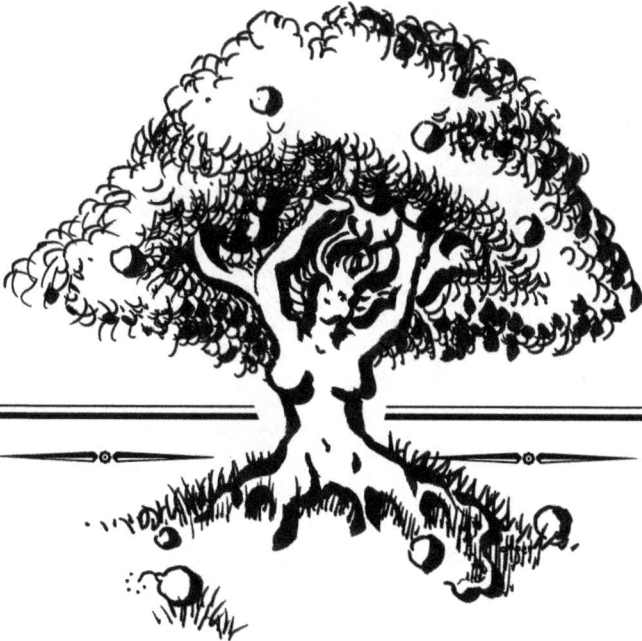

Try Everything

MACROBIOTIC DIET

At first, when I was trying to keep my cancer secret, I would cringe at these words, "Oh, I am so sorry to hear your news." Invariably, some advice would follow that I would not even listen to, being already so irritated at the first part of the sentence. But, I was too weak to fight and, I had to hear the whole thing. I learned to relax, swallow my pride, and let the advice roll in.

Angela, my friend and neighbor, learned of my "predicament." We'd been friends for years and both participated in the kids' carpool to ballet classes and performances at the Pennsylvania Ballet. Oh my god, it was big in our lives! Both of my children were dancers with the Metropolitan Ballet Studio in Cheltenham. Every December, the children would try out for positions in The Nutcracker Suite. They had to train a lot. The carpool community had about it the magical excitement of the rosy-cheeked, dancing, spirit of Christmas.

"I know a guy who tried a special diet," Angela avoided saying he had cancer. Totally avoided the word. How smart. The word hurt.

"Okay." I was still irritated but too weak, and I loved Angela.

"And, he is still alive," she would continue to push.

"Okay." I did not fight.

"Do you want to know about it?"

"Sure." I tried my best.

"OK, then," said Angela. "I will get you the contact information of his dietitian. You know, he was given one year, but it's been like seven years and he is still alive."

I agreed. That was the strongest argument: being alive. Then, for the first time, I saw that as the total and only sense. Do what has been shown to keep people alive. It does not matter how crazy, illogical, irrational, or unscientific. What's science, anyway, if not the ability to observe and analyze those observations?

Soon, Angela passed me the information of this cancer dietitian and wrote a letter to introduce me to her. Finally, we met. Her name was Marilyn. She was all about the macrobiotic diet. At first the price seemed too high, and I argued with her a little bit, but she was stern: initial consultations would cost something and then I would be able to consult with her for several weeks. I really battled with the idea that I had to pay so much money, even though I now think of it as worth every cent. She was my first out-of-pocket expense. This divergence from traditional medicine represented another step towards accepting responsibility for my own life, setting aside the comfortable passivity of being "taken care of"

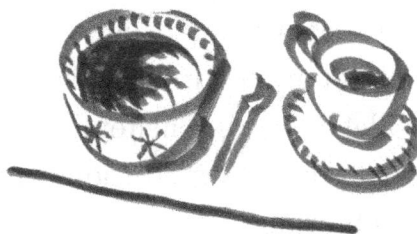

by a supposedly omnipotent system. I contacted Marilyn at the end of March, and had my first session in the beginning of June of 2009.

I fell out of the circle of paid services, and my feeling of normalcy was shaken when I disobeyed the projected voices of the mainstream majority telling me not to try something for what an insurance company would not pay. Now I think this "insurance company rule" is actually our fear ruling our ability to rationally look at the reality and decide on our own what is good for us and what is not.

When I paid my first out-of pocket expense, my first $250 dollars, a meager amount in the face of all those future travels, vaccines and other remedies thrown in the face of the beast, I felt extremely empowered. I played cards with fate; it wanted me to know how serious I was. But I was trying to choose my games wisely. The moment I let go of this $250 something changed.

I loved it. This food made sense! I felt light and strong. My yin and yang were calculated and harmonized. The non-dairy rule was more familiar to me than no-shade veggies one but, overall, I liked and understood the meal plan. There were so many Japanese products whose names I did not know that, at first, my head spun. However, Marilyn was near and available for advice. Plus, I was shopping at Essene Market, the fantastic macrobiotic store in Philadelphia. It was super cool. I loved shiitake mushrooms, arame, hijiki. Kombu (sea vegetables), shoyu (sauce), azuki beans, umeboshi plums (salty!), dried daikon, sweet rice, miso soups all the time

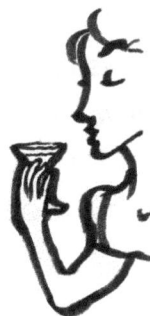

and salmon for strength. My first successful dish was azuki beans with daikon and hijiki. It smelled like fish, because I didn't wash the hijiki long enough, but I mastered it, after a while, and everyone liked it. I took a class on cooking sea veggies, and loved it. The diet was time consuming, of course, but Angela's story about the man with cancer who was still alive was a strong antidote to laziness. I wanted to live!

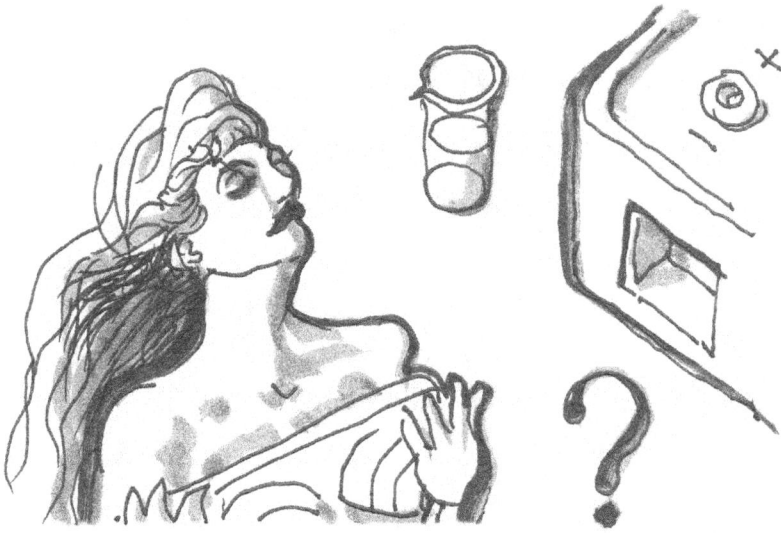

SOVIET MYSTERY APPARATUS

My father is an extremely skeptical, extremely logical man, and yet he spent several hundred dollars for a mysterious Russian apparatus without the slightest understanding of how it could possibly work. "Why not try everything?" he said. He sent this device along with my mother when she came to help. That meant that she had to be the one to read all the very unclear and mysterious instructions.

The apparatus itself was packaged with an instructional booklet and several CDs. The instructions were a mess. My mom called my aunt, the apparatus proponent, twice a day to ask her questions. They were both very frustrated. My mom at the fact the aunt is not giving her the clear answers, and my aunt at my mom for being so slow. Finally, my mom decided that she had figured it out enough, and started using it. I don't know how I should even describe it but let me try. When the apparatus was turned on for 'input,' it made a slight spaceship buzz. My mom had figured out, with my aunt and from the instructions, to hover the apparatus over a jar of my morning urine for a while. At this point, it would be considered charged. Then, I would turn the apparatus in the "out" position and hover it over my chest. I used this device every day. Who's to say it didn't cure my cancer?

CHAPTER 16
Cancer Kumbaya

By then, I had already heard from friends and doctors about clinical trials. I did not know what to expect, but it sounded magical. I wanted to get into one. I trusted the hospital I'd already enrolled with, because it belonged to the University of Pennsylvania Hospital System. There actually, also, is the University of Pennsylvania Hospital, which had separate facilities but I hoped that, since these two belonged to the same system, they would be identical in terms of clinical trials.

When it was time for the chemo, Dr. Mayor told me not to worry because the oncologist who was going to prescribe my treatment was an excellent doctor.

"She is great," he said. "Make an appointment with her. My part is done, but you can call me anytime."

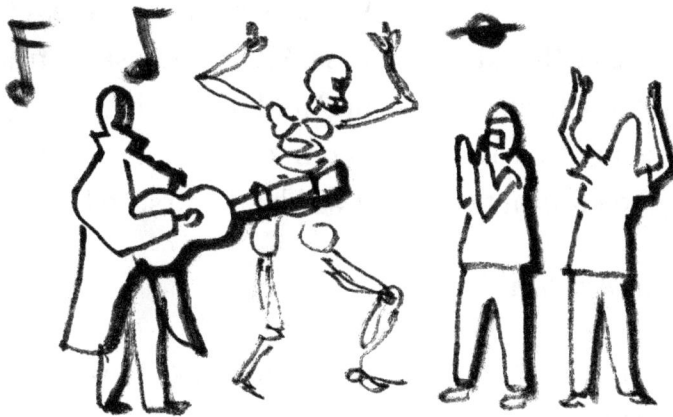

I arranged an appointment with the oncologist and bided my time by looking into the possibility of clinical trials at Fox Chase. The doctor I met with said that the only clinical trial he knew about included Avastin, a drug blocking growth of blood vessels to a tumor. Because I had had a stroke, I could not and should not want to participate in this trial. As far as this doctor was concerned, I was out of luck. This is when my husband cried and stopped taking notes, and this was the last time I asked him to accompany me.

In a way, this chain of events was a stroke of luck. When the time came for my appointment with the oncologist Dr. Mayor had recommended, I asked my friend Lynn to go with me. This appointment would be one of the decisive points in the development of my story, which started to take unexpected turns. The oncologist would lie to me, thinking that I was too naïve to grasp the real situation, and my friend Lynn would help me see through it. I desperately wanted to get into any clinical trial.

"You seem to be part of the University of Pennsylvania. Do you share clinical trials with them?" I asked.

"Yes, of course. Not to worry. We have the same access to clinical trials as they do. Of course. We run the same trials. If there are any trials, believe me" and her cheerful arrogant confidence made us ashamed of ourselves, almost "if there are any good clinical trials, you will be the first to know."

"How about Avastin?"

"Hmm. Yeah. For that, hmm, you would have to wait. And, besides, you may not qualify."

"And, about clinical trials," she said."Do you know that you might even end up in the branch that does not get the new drug? Wouldn't that be terrifying?"

Later, my friend Lynn and I agreed that, in spite of the doctor's assurances about access to clinical trials, her real agenda was as a salesperson of good ol' traditional chemo. Everything she said was geared to reinforce this single course of default treatment. She gave us a tour of the "wonderful facility," a bunch of recliner chairs with people dozing off, some with no hair, some young, but all with that attitude of heroism that hospitals encourage to soothe the real fight in a patient, the fight to find a real cure! I wanted a life-saving solution, not a face to put on while I settled for a stop-gap standard product line of treatments.

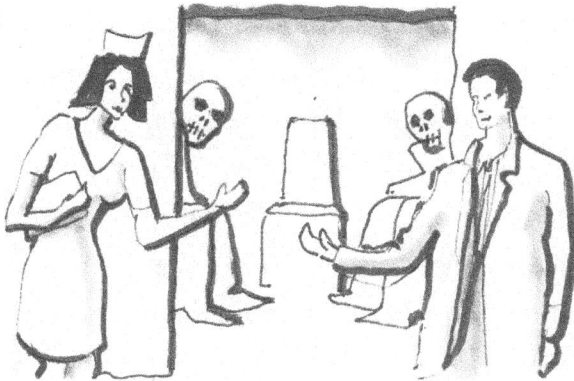

Every chemical in use for chemotherapy had been in use for twenty or thirty years, and none of them promised more than an average of three years of survival. These came with a free paper attitude, just like a Burger King crown, and each patient was expected to be giddy as a child to get to sing the catchy "cancer Kumbaya."

But I was tired of looking, and so the highly recommended oncologist masterfully manipulated me and, before I knew what had happened, I was being admitted for the standard therapy, even though it seemed stunningly awful.

STANDARD CARE CYTOTOXIC DRUGS

I was advised to use the "standard of care combination of old, cytotoxic drugs that break cell division." All dividing cells die while the drug is administered. The premise is that, since cancer cells divide very rapidly, they will be the ones that are killed. A curious mind would probably ask: Are there other types of dividing cells in the body? The answer is: Yes. What about them? Will they be killed too? The answer is: Yes. What are these cells that are dividing, besides the cancerous cells? The answer is: immune cells including T-lymphocytes, B-lymphocytes, dendritic cells, platelets. They are the product of dividing pre-T-lymphocytes, pre-B-lymphocyte, pre-dendritic cells, pre-platelets. These progenitor cells are not the fully functional immune cells capable of killing bacteria (B-lymphocytes) or killing cells, invaded with viruses and cancer (T-lymphocytes). They are progenitor cells, living in the bone marrow and lymph nodes, developing into mature warrior cells.

And, yes, since the drug does not know which of the dividing cells are cancerous, it just blindly attaches to spindles or the DNA in all dividing cells it encounters, and these cells are obliterated. For peritoneal cancer, they use the same drugs they do for ovarian cancer: platinum-based cisplatin or carboplatin, and a more generic and more widely used drug called taxol.

✛═┠╸ CHAPTER 17 ✛═┠╸

Chemo

On April 21st, 2009, I gave up looking for clinical trials and surrendered to the chorus of voices threatening me with death. But, before that, I went to the salon and asked them for a very short haircut. I tried to joke with the hair dresser about being a cancer patient donating it hair for wigs instead of losing it to chemotherapy, but she was horrified and did not say a word. She cut off my hair in a silent horror. I should have been more careful with my jokes.

I stopped joking when I arrived at the hospital. It all looked so casual, as if they were not injecting deadly stuff into people's bodies. Nurses surrounded me singing their Kumbaya "you-gonna-be-ok-here-is-our-wonderful-nutrition-specailist-patients-love-her" while they dragged me around and between and through the patient-heroes. They found a free recliner chair, sat me in it, and connected me to the IV. It still felt like a thing that had to be done urgently, a decision that could have been of the utmost importance. And it still felt like a lie: a last meal before execution, a meaningless indulgence.

The infusion of the drug taxol took something like four hours: nothing dramatic.

"You will lose your hair, Ms. Gutkina."

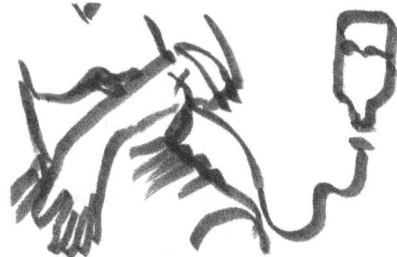

"Are you sure?"

"Oh, yeah. No doubt about it."

I left sad, unsure if I had done the right thing. There was something wrong about this place, this hospital. Dr. Mendax was aloof and overconfident. Dr. Mayor, who I thought would be taking care of my treatments, just passed all authority back to the same oncologist who I didn't trust. It was all slightly weird, not personal, not on target, very removed from me and my many needs and questions. I already knew to look for alternatives when anything felt weird. I decided to go to UPenn. It took me a lot of courage. I thought that this Institute was too good for me and that they would never take me. Why did I think that? I don't know but I know that I am not alone thinking like that. There would be other patients who would not "dare" to go to the best hospital in town for the same reason. They did not feel they were worth it. They stayed with their under-performing doctors and died.

Being "shy" in that fundamental way, I asked a worthier proxy to help me climb the "hospital ladder." A friend of Gosha's, Dr. Tolik, had kept promising that he would set up an appointment for me with Dr. Howe, who was the best gynecologic oncologist in Philadelphia. Dr. Tolik kept promising to call Dr. Howe, at UPenn, but he never actually did.

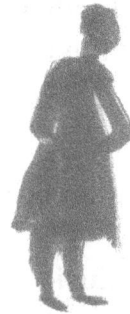

Since then, I have made a rule not to wait for someone if he does not immediately do what he has promised. He and his wife are still good friends, but I felt bitter about it at the time. I suppose I should have called Dr. Howe, myself.

I should have rushed there the very first day I knew about my diagnosis. Instead, I waited for my friend, Dr. Tolik, to make that call for me!

Something in the attitude of the overconfident Dr. Mendax scared me and propelled me to action. So I had to collect all my courage and make an appointment myself. I called UPenn and asked for an appointment with Dr. Howe. They asked me to send over my reports, which I did. I got the appointment very easily, in a couple of days. I did not expect that. It was easy and fast. There was one receptionist who gave me trouble but, by then, I was immune to receptionists' powers, and I made it through her. I talked to other people in the office, and they seemed unusually nice.

The difference was radical, between UPenn and all other hospitals I'd seen. With the exception of the one receptionist, the staff was incredible. Instead of trying to scare patients with the grandeur of their power, they asked real questions and made genuine small talk, and tried to make you feel better any way they could. They did this skillfully and sincerely. I was shocked by what Dr. Howe had to say.

"We have a clinical trial for your peritoneal cancer. It's a promising new drug."

"Oh?!"

"Wait. Did you already start chemo?"

"Yes. A couple days ago."

"Oops. Sorry. You don't qualify."

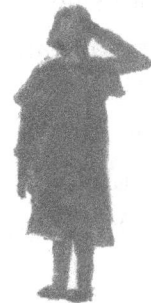

"WHY??!!!"

"Oh, well, because you've already started the chemo."

"Wait. Dr. Howe. My oncologist told me that she, I mean her hospital, and you share the same clinical trials."

"No."

"She assured me."

"I am sorry. That information is wrong."

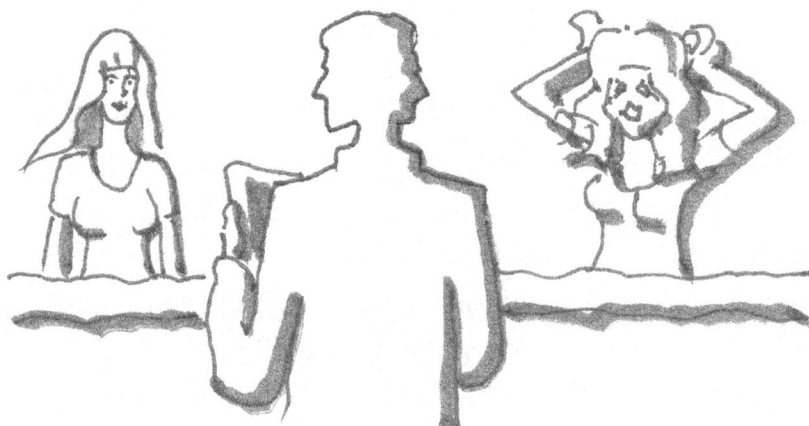

" . . . . "

"I can suggest that you finish your treatment there, and then you can come to us. Say, when you relapse."

I was frustrated beyond words! I realized that Dr. Mendax had LIED. But what was worse, I now had no chance of getting into UPenn's clinical trial and had to stick to treatments where I was guaranteed to relapse, very soon. I was so frustrated. I blamed Dr. Tolik for dragging his feet. I blamed myself for not taking charge. I was devastated and angry. But, who said it was going to be easy?!

CHAPTER 18

Doctors and Doctors

Professionals can be divided into two categories: fake and real. Some doctors would celebrate their power to hide their ignorance, and look down on those heroes, those five percent who are trying to change the status quo. I know one fake doctor who called a real one a charlatan. This fake doctor laughed at the notion of dendritic cells and cancer immunotherapy, in 2011! This was after the discovery of dendritic cells had been awarded the Nobel Prize! I am very angry at this particular fake doctor at one regional Philadelphia hospital.

I was accompanying my friend's mom to her appointment. The woman was diagnosed with leukemia and was undergoing aggressive chemotherapy and radiation under his, as I later found out, sinister care. By then, friends considered me an expert in dealing with cancer situations, and I was there for support and questions. I was still a bit naïve, and did not know the extent of animosity and aggravation that my quiet question, "What do you think of immunotherapy?" would stir. He yelled at me, "Charlatans!" I was still trying to make conversation. He yelled louder and louder, spitting out specious facts with every angry phrase.

What a jealous brat! Yes, it was jealousy—violent and ugly—the jealousy of someone without talent or creativity. I have seen it many times and I recognize its manifestations, very well. When, later, I created my company, I heard the same voices, "She is crazy. What she did is nothing. She needs to be punished. I am the real owner." Ogh. I know this jealousy all too well, now. I was angry and devastated, every time it happened. I heard "you are nothing," as soon as I started to see the fruits of my creation. I heard it from my partners, who wanted to own it and push me out and run it, from my father, from my husband, from many other dear people who might even claim they love me. But, in the grip of jealousy, they are reduced to irrational hostility.

This doctor from Jefferson University Hospital shared a story with me, a supposedly triumphant one, of how the "charlatans" were let go. One of them even became a regulatory consultant, a non-practicing physician. "That is what you get if you are a charlatan," he said. It is sad that he needed others to be persecuted in order to feel legitimate. I knew the real story about these real doctors. I knew a woman who had been their former patient. She has been cancer free for fifteen years, an eternity! I met this woman at a meeting of the Sandy Ovarian foundation, where I was proselytizing my dendritic vaccine, and she told me she had been treated with one fifteen years before.

"Where? How?"

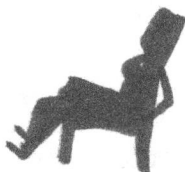 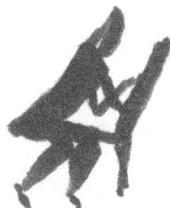

She gave me the names of her two doctors: "But they are not working there anymore. One of them is a regulatory consultant somewhere in Jersey. They had troubles, you know." She could not tell me anything else, but she was here, alive, on this Earth, going on with her life, more than a decade after her diagnosis. That was all I needed to know.

In the care of the fake doctor, my friend's mother died within two months. Her chemotherapy was not curing her cancer, but was effectively killing her. The fake doctor's failure did not effect him professionally because it was an accepted standard of care, an expected type of failure. "PEOPLE DIE BECAUSE IT IS CANCER AND THEY ARE SUPPOSED TO." This concept has become an accepted excuse for not trying to think creatively, for not trying to save each, individual patient.

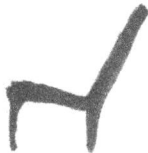

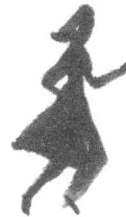

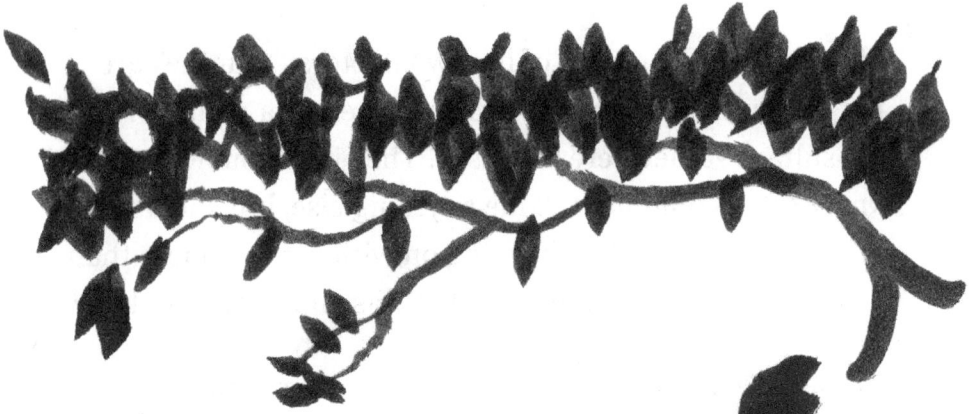

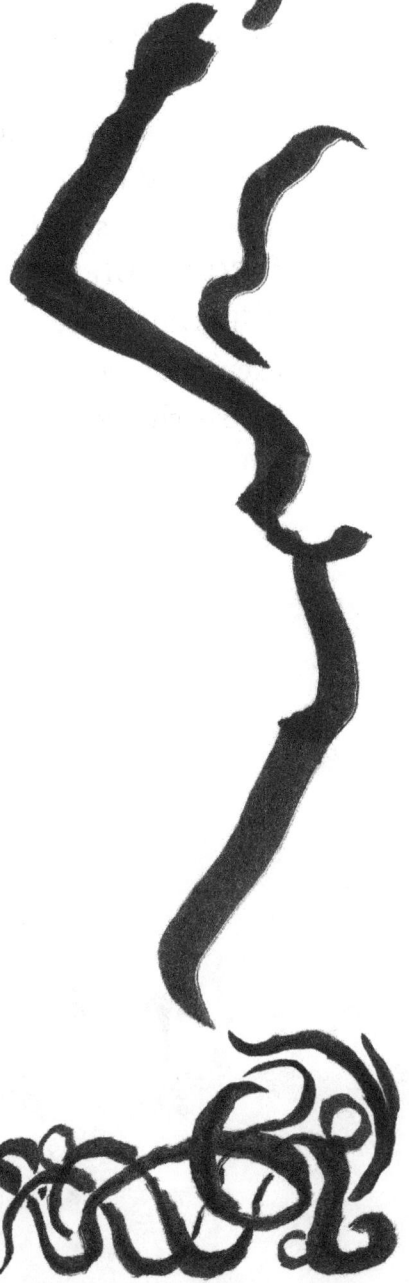

PART III

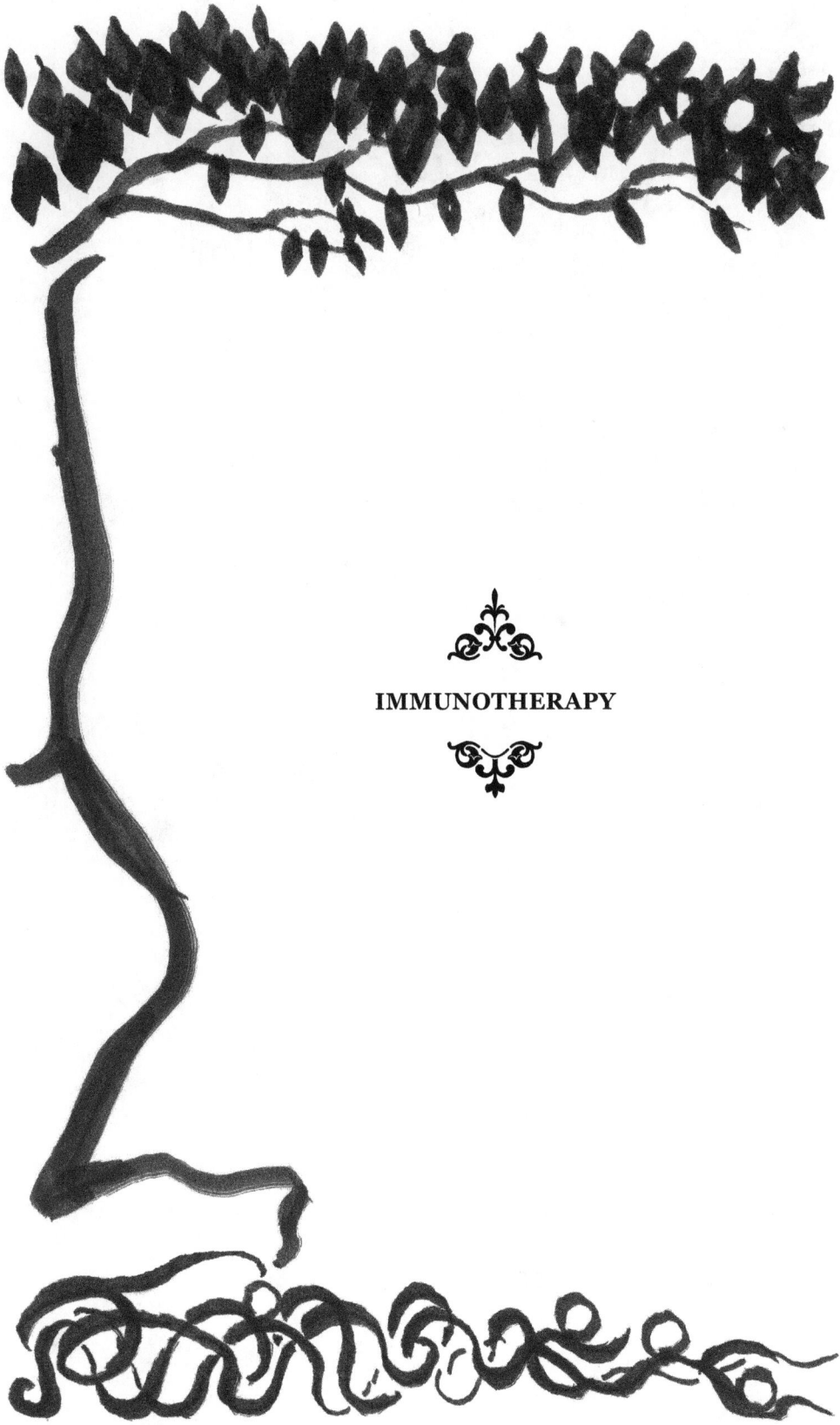

IMMUNOTHERAPY

CHAPTER 19

The Call

⁕ I ⁕

"Hi, Anechka. You must get out of bed and go to Russia. Can you do it tomorrow?"

I almost hung up. "Who is this?"

"Anechka! Don't hang up. We were THERE. With Aleksandr Sergeyvich. I know what I am talking about. It was horrible. Believe me. But now he is fine. Seven years. He jumped out of it. Vika told me about you."

Vika was a friend with whom I'd been recently reconciled.

"No problem. Anechka, what are you doing right now? For example, are you lying in bed?"

She sounded kind but I sensed it was the fake kindness of a manipulator. The question was a mine ready to explode in the next sentence. If I avoided stepping on it, she would detonate it, anyway.

"Aghmmm. Yeah...I don't know..."

"It's probably okay. But how are you feeling?" and, before I had a chance to answer,"Well, of course you might feel a little bad but... and you might lie down sometimes... YOU SHOULD NOT BE IN BED RIGHT NOW."

"Aghmm."

"What? Can't hear you!! Why are in bed? Vika told me you feel well. You can take a plane, right?"

"I don't know…"

"I know. Vika told me. Anechka, you are doing all right. BUT BE AWARE. You might have a false feeling that you are all right. Please don't trust it. You are dying unless you do something."

"But I am doing chemo, what else can I do?"

"Oh, no! CHEMO?! You are insane. Chemo is the worst thing you could have done!"

I was trembling, already, on my end of the line. At this point, she realized she had pushed too hard and retreated into her earlier, sweet and kind voice.

"I mean, Anechka. We spent years studying cancer. Me and Aleksandr Sergeyvich know that chemo is breeding resistant cells. You understand?"

"Perhaps."

"Of course you don't. You were not doing any science for years, right?"

"Right, but I…"

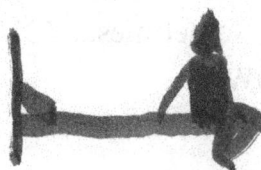
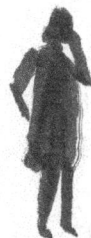

"Never mind. I know. Resistance. All they do with chemo is selection for resistant clones."

I was almost crying.

"OK never mind. You did what you did. But we, Aleksandr Sergeyvich and I, we knew how fast these cancer clones are growing. Every day they multiply. And we knew we should be in a hurry. And we flew to Russia IN EIGHT DAYS AFTER THE DIAGNOSIS. EIGHT DAYS. How long have you known?"

"About a month."

"Oh my God. But don't worry. Get up and go to Mitya."

I had a feeling my friend Vika had been helping me, behind my back.I figured the channel she had made this connection was through my brother's wife, since my brother knew all about my predicament. Vika must have arranged this conversation with Dr. Natalyia Nikolaevna Petrov, an activist scientist.

"Aleksandr Sergeyvich is fine, and you will be too," she declared. "Just get out of your gruesome bed RIGHT NOW and GO TO RUSSIA."

I knew that Aleksandr Sergeyevich was Natalia Nikolaevna's husband, and they liked to be referred to in the Russian tradition. They had been working and living in America for twenty years, but still kept a lot of Russian attitudes. Natalia Nikolaevna Petrov was a cancer researcher, a cell biologist studying the resistance of cancer cells to drugs among other things related to cancer.

So, of course, I did not hang up. I was already falling for Natalia Nikolaevna Petrov's energy, knowledge and the persuasive opinion of a top-notch cancer researcher. She seemed to know what I should be doing, but was careful sometimes when she sensed she was pushing too hard. She had the experience and intuition of a leader, and knew when to push and when to back off. But, most of all, she was trying to save me in earnest and spent a lot of time and energy doing that. She was manipulating and leading me for my own good. She wanted to save my life.

⇢ II ⇠

"What, you are doing chemo? But it is horrible! Of course it is your choice but, when Aleksandr Sergeyvich got sick, we immediately went to Russia. We did surgery, then the dendritic vaccine and no chemo. It is seven years now, and he is fine. He only has one lung, but he is fine."

They told me their story in detail. This is one of the stories people tell all the time, and when we became friends with the Petrovs later, I heard this story many times. I didn't mind. It was a trademark family story. Aleksandr Sergeyevich used to be a heavy smoker. Natalia Nikolaevna was concerned, and warned him that one day he would get lung cancer. "And you know, one day I found out that I did have lung cancer, and walked into the room and I told her: Natasha, You were right, this day is now. I have lung cancer."

Natalaya Nikolaevna continued:

"Anechka, we did not wait another moment. They told us to

get ready for the hospice, because they would not operate on him. And, we knew that we should do everything we could before he gets too sick to travel."

"From then on, we sprang into action and we were in Russia eight days after the diagnosis. We were heading to Mitya for his dendritic vaccine. The Petrovs knew a lot of professional people on both continents. They knew a surgeon in Saint Petersburg who was able to operate and remove one lung. It was a difficult decision, I guess, as are all important decisions, but it was necessary to make it. After waking up from anesthesia, Aleksandr Sergeyevich was gasping for air. We were not sure if he would need oxygen. We decided he would rather adjust."

"And I adjusted," Aleksandr continued. "Now, when people ask me how I feel, I say: 'Imagine you are climbing a high mountain. Like you're breathing the mountain air. That's me.'" When he talks a lot, he starts to breathe heavily.

His wife resumed, "We did not even save the tissue for the antigen preparation. I was so shocked that I just stood there like a fool, and watched the tissue go to trash! Aleksandr Sergeyvich had several injections. It was hard. It was right after surgery. He was shaking." Both Dr. Petrovs were quiet for a moment. "But hey, it was seven years ago. Seven!"

"I jumped out of it." Aleksandr Sergeyvich sounded like a teenager who accomplished a difficult board trick. "I jumped out. I am free."

Listening to this amazing story, I realized I had to do the same thing. What was the name? Mitya? Dendritic vaccine?

Soon I made the connection with Dr. Mitya, whom I call Dr. Dmitry. Mitya is his former student's friendly nickname. I chose a more formal, appropriate version. Soon after, I dialed Dr. Dmitry's cell phone. He immediately agreed to see me.

"When are you available?"

"Any time."

"Are you in the city next week, for example?" I asked.

"Yes. I am always in the city. But, you need to bring the tumor with you."

"What do you mean?"

"Do you have tumor tissue saved anywhere? Frozen in a freezer at your hospital?"

"I guess, 'No.' I don't know. I guess I have to ask."

"For the dendritic vaccine, we need an antigen, which is the tumor tissue."

"I did not ask them to store it..."

"They must have done pathology analysis."

"They must have... I don't know. Yeah, I have the report."

"You need to call them and get me some tissue. Better if it's frozen. But I know they probably should have the paraffin slides at least. At least these. Bring me something, if you can."

I was starting to get it. To develop my own dendritic vaccine, I would need to have my own tumor cells as an antigen.

Even though I was a biochemist, I had not worked in biology for thirteen years and it took me a while to understand how dendritic vaccines work. At first, I just trusted Dr. Dmitry. His success with Dr. Petrov and his track record of treating patients with glioma, were all the evidence I needed. I did not have time, back then, to study dendritic vaccines. Instead, I was making calls to the hospital to get my tissue, and getting ready to go to Russia with my cancer tissue samples. I called the Patients Records Departments first.

"Can I get some tissue?"

They could not understand what I was saying.

"Let me transfer you to the Pathology Department Head."

"Okay."

"The Head is out of town... You need to call this number."

"Okay."

I called the number and explained that I need the tumor tissue left from my surgery.

"How many days have passed? We may not have it. Can you call in a couple of days, when a guy who is responsible for the tissue will be back?"

"Yes, but could you make a note that I want you not to throw away my tissue in the

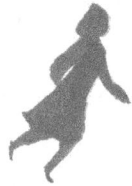

meanwhile? It is very important to me."

"Ma'am, I don't know what you are talking about. Just call this number. Bye-bye."

⇥ III ⇤

Day after day, I was trying to get information about whether the hospital had any tissue stored. I spent hours on the phone being transferred between people who were nice and people who weren't.

"At least, tell me where my paraffin slides are."

"Oh, paraffin slides. We sent them to Fox Chase for evaluation."

"And?"

After numerous calls this news:"I believe they lost them, Ms. Gutkina."

Nice. They lost my slides. I had no antigen for the vaccine. The Petrovs did not have an antigen, either, and the vaccine still worked, however.

I dialed the Petrovs'.

"I don't have the tumor tissue for the antigen. What shall I do?"

"No tissue? Wow. What are they thinking about? Of course they never heard about the immunotherapy. Don't even mention it to them." In a year, the dendritic cell discovery would be awarded the Nobel Prize.

"Nothing," I admitted.

"Well. We did not have it either, I told you." Natalya Nikolaevna told me the story again, how they flew to Saint Petersburg immediately after they knew Dr. Petrov had lung cancer. "They gave him 2 months! They were putting him in the hospice! And we said, 'No. We are going to Russia.'"

Dr. Natalya Petrov told me, again, how they went to a Saint Petersburg hospital to see the surgeon, an old friend of theirs. He cut the effected lung out. "Just cut it out," she said. "I was there in the operating room. It was too much. I was all confused."

I did not mind hearing the story again and again.

She went on: "I was so confused that I did not even think about saving the tumor. It all went so quickly."

"And then how did you prepare the vaccine?"

"Without the antigen."

"And it still worked, apparently."

"Anechka. We had faith in our protocol and Mitya and the technology, and it saved us. It will save you, too. It is a real thing."

"So, you were missing the antigen, but the vaccine worked without it?" I asked her once again.

"Yes. Just go there as soon as you can."

"I am surprised you can't locate your tumor though," she added with a slightly commanding tone, as if she was disappointed with my performance. She used to run a big lab in Russia and this commanding attitude never really left her, even after many years on the bench at several US universities. I would have been embarrassed at my poor performance with finding my own tumor antigen, if it was a different setting, but I did not have to care about my impression on anybody, anymore. I just thanked her and moved on to more important tasks. I called Dr. Dmitry:

"I can't find the tumor anywhere. Can I come without it?"

"Not even slides?" he asked.

"Not even slides. They lost it."

"OK," Dr. Dmitry said. "Come without. We'll try."

Gosha booked me the ticket to Saint Petersburg, right away. It was about a week after chemo, more like several days. I still had my hair, however, I expected to lose it pretty soon.

THE SECRET SOCIETY OF CANCER

I was getting a lot of calls from the old friends who had disappeared from my life years ago. At first I was so deep in my desperation that I did not want to share anyting with anybody, and just wanted to be left alone. True friends, like Vika, my college buddy, kept calling.

One day I gave in and called Vika and we started to communicate. Vika's husband died from cancer several years ago.

We talked about that for a while. People whose lives were affected by cancer are different in their attitudes towards each other – towards other people affected by cancer. It is a society of the closest bonds, the tightest connections, stronger than any secret society; it is like a brotherhood of early Christian knights, connected by virtue, loving their members but secretive to the outsiders. There is no shame in telling each other's stories in this No Secret Cancer Society. And we shared ours.

Vika's husband Lev tried to cure himself from his cancer. A smart and experienced cancer researcher, he had his own ideas about the nature of the beast. So he refused to undergo chemotherapy, knowing as a researcher that cytotoxic drugs harm the immune system and other systems in the body. He was juicing and taking some alternative non-toxic remedies that were supposed to help. When I knew him, he was already sick, but full of energy and a desire to develop his idea into a technology. Lev was a cytologist working with cancer cells. He was observing changes in a cancer cell's chromosomes, and in the age of computers, he wanted to create an automated protocol for recognition of all these aberrations and abnormalities. He contacted Gosha, and they were working on these ideas for a while. He wanted to name his future protocol "Stella" to honor his beloved boss Stella, who died from cancer a couple years before that. Doctor Stella never underwent chemotherapy either, and relied on macrobiotic diet and alternative methods, I am not sure which ones. Lev was going to Russia for a treatment that was suggested to him by a Russian scientist. As far as I remember, they were injecting cytokines or a

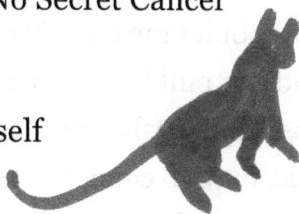

particular cytokine.

Unfortunately it did not help. Lev died soon after we were discussing his idea. I still feel very guilty that Gosha and I took the responsibility of developing it into a business, and did not fulfill the promise. It would have been a nice thing to have for his wife and his child after he was gone. The guys wanted to drive their business idea themselves, and did not let me and Vika in. Between the two of them they did not pull it off while Lev was still capable. The time was lost, and Gosha could not do it alone when Lev started to succumb to cancer. When I asked about how things were going Gosha would say:"OK. We are thinking." Thinking and doing nothing led to failure. I feel bad that I transferred my responsibility and the good intentions did not materialize.

Lev and Mr. Petrov, were going to Russia for cancer treatments that they pretty much invented for themselves, at the same time. Mr. Petrov has gone a different way than Lev.

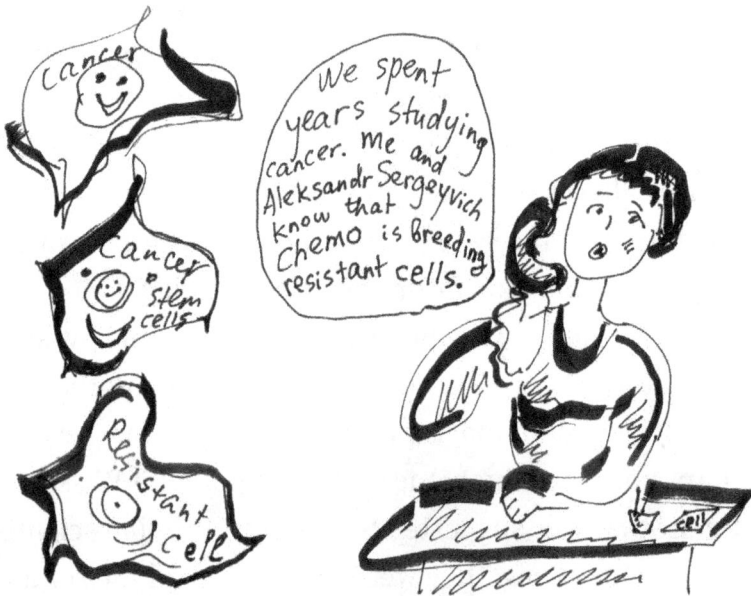

His treatment invention proved to be the better one, and he was still alive, 7 years after his diagnosis, and cancer free all this time. Lev has been gone for several years now.

Vika told me the story calmly, as a matter of fact. We were having a lot of conversations those days, I think we were on the phone constantly. I had a chance to say how sorry I was that Lev was gone. She took it very gracefully, not a hint of bitterness. She was there to help me. She told me she was crying for me all the time.

The crying notion made me uncomfortable. I loved Vika even more now, because I saw how deep her love was for me. When we were in college, we had a lot in common, mostly our mixed Jewish-Russian upbringing, and a genius Daddy in the family, the constant background to everything we were doing in life. I think she loved me back then for no reason, the same way that she loved our other friends. Her capacity for love and devotion is enormous. She thinks I am a genius too, because of one episode in the chemistry exam.

For some reason, I was one of very few people in the class who grasped the material. It was strange to observe how other people were just not getting how entropies, enthalpies and Gibbs energies were connected to manifest order, chaos and the transitions between them. So after I was done with my exam work, I went over to help out my friend Masha. Masha is very smart, but this chemistry test was something she seemed to be about to fail, her eyes were wide open with the fear of failing the test. I quickly sketched some answers for her. And this is where Vika became my absolute fan. Since then not only I am enjoying her love, but her conviction that I am the real genius. This is great if someone thinks you are genius! Vika was suddenly there, ready to help. She insisted that I talk to Mr. and Mrs. Petrov and do the same thing that they did to stay alive after the horrible diagnosis.

"They did not do chemo," Vika told me. "They are totally against chemo. Talk to them."

I was tortured whether to do the chemo or not. From one side, I heard all the voices that chemo kills. However Lev's story showed that his trips to an alternative clinic to Mexico and his resistance to get chemo did not help.

I was torn. But I decided to do chemo and everything that alternative methods could offer.

**DEDICATION &
CERTIFICATION OF
THANKS TO:**

*Elena & Sergei
Kurenov*

**ANNA THANKS YOU FOR
YOUR KIND SUPPORT!**

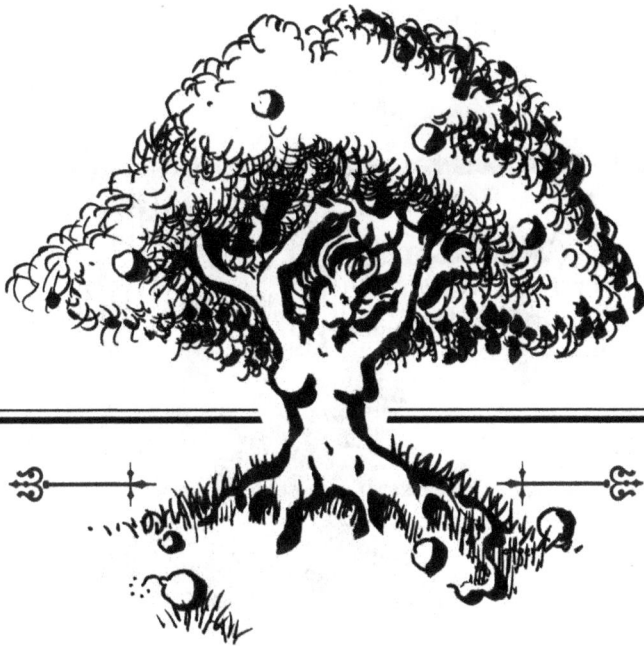

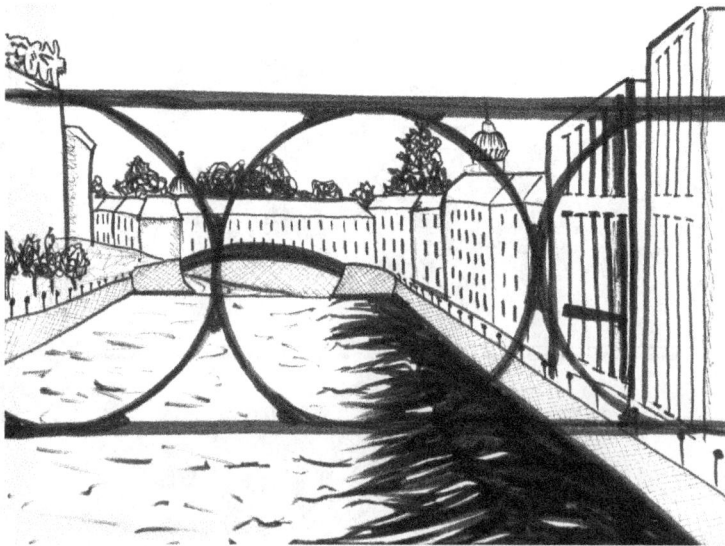

CHAPTER 20
Russia

My first trip to Russia was rather dramatic because I felt like a weak person, a dying patient in need of attention and protection, vulnerable in every way. I needed to have my own macrobiotic food, I was shooting anti-coagulation medicine into my thigh every day, and I was out of my comfy death bed with its view of the big maple tree.

I completely cut out meat and all dairy from my diet. I ate beans, rice and fish. I took several little bags of grain to Russia with me. My dad and his second wife Natasha had prepared to cook macrobiotic for me when I came to stay with them in Saint Petersburg. I also bought several containers to carry food with me because I treated everything that was not macrobiotic and pure as poison, and would not touch the airplane food. I was carrying my food containers with a sense of proud importance that my disease gave me. I proudly booked the tickets with the vegetarian food option, that gave an additional boost, and I think I am going to try other exclusive options next time I fly. Food is a great tool if you want to feel special!

Thus equipped, I came to Saint Petersburg and went to draw blood for the dendritic vaccine. A dear friend of mine, Masha, arranged for my blood to be drawn at her research institute. Masha was always a kind friend. I could always rely on her. Masha's mother rushed to help, immediately. She was a surgeon at a Special Medical Academy, historically one of the best hospitals in the city. She arranged

my appointment with yet another oncologist, a doctor in
the Academy, whom she trusted. I was still hungry to hear
a second opinion. Everything had happened so quickly
and I was not sure I was doing the right thing. I wouldn't
have much time in Saint Petersburg. I had to be back in
Philadelphia in a week for the another round of chemo.

So in Russia I was supposed to do my first vaccine with Dr.
Dmitry. He was the reason I came back. He was my Russia.

I trusted Dr. Dmitry completely and blindly. It was
somewhat easy because I had no choice, but it was easy
also because he was a man of purpose and determination
beyond anything I have ever seen before in my life. His
respect for a human life was at the center of his existence.
This was his unabashed stand. He stood up for life.

He was formed by a tragedy. His wife died of
cancer, and this man, humble and shy, became
a stubborn warrior against cancer. For many
years he attacked cancer from left and right. But mostly it
was dendritic cells and T-cells. Twenty some years ago the
establishment frowned upon him, just like they frowned
upon all those "dendritic people" all over the world. Nobody
took him seriously perhaps. He did not have enough money
for his studies, because it was the rampaging Russian
nineties, cruel to the weak and removed from the luxuries
of scientific research. He continued on.

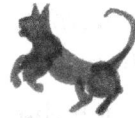

One of the cancer institutes however "allowed" Dr. Dmitry
in. I am just imagining him going to place after place and
the looks that people of power gave him, a look of the gate-
keeper to a possibility they had no idea existed. A "who is

this?" look. I imagine it took a lot of perseverance from Dr. Dmitry to press on his dendritic vaccine. And I imagine how much courage it should have taken for a person of power to let somebody like him in. And work together.

A serendipitous circle of friends included my best friend from high school, Ira. Her dad was the person of power who let Dr. Dmitry in. The laws of existence continued to unravel in a magical way.

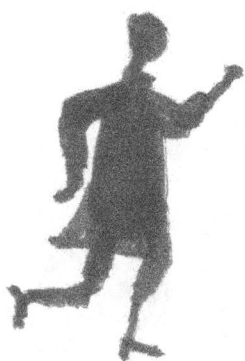

CHAPTER 21
Ode to Wigs

It was April, about a week after chemo, and my short hair would begin to fall out in about a week. The comb was full every time I brushed my hair. I could see my skin more and more. The view of me in the mirror without hair was terrifyingly ugly. If I had not seen multiple pictures of cancer patients, bald from chemo, I would have been crushed, embarrassed beyond belief, almost destroyed. The media replication of the cancer patient image was a very useful thing for me. I think it is the horror of the unknown that keeps us repeating cycles of behavior, even if they don't work. On the other hand, if the fear of death is greater than the horror of the unknown, we can do things differently.

Before my entire head of hair fell out, my dad and I went to a wig store and we bought a short wig. It was kind of a strange color, but I couldn't stand for it to be completely natural, for some reason. I chose one that was a kind of copper red. Then a friend noted that this is the favorite color Russian women use to dye their hair. True! I didn't think about it, then. Later, I decided to play with my image, since I had an opportunity to do whatever I wanted. I did not even have to dye the hair, or grow it. I could just buy a new wig.

I decided to become a blonde. Nobody knew I had cancer so, when I appeared at one of my meetings in a wig, people complimented me on my new hair style. This was the most successful period on my life! That day, with my dad, we tried several wigs. I felt the power of blondeness. I started a business, effortlessly. I was making a lot of connections in the business community and everybody liked me and felt my power, the power of a tall blonde woman. That was fantastic! But that would be a little later, so bear with me for a while.

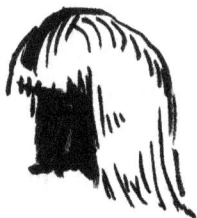

I am very grateful that my dad was completely cool and casual about the wig and other sorts of details. It was very important to keep busy, not to get emotional and waste precious time thinking about how people would react and what could have been done but was not. If something or somebody turned out to be a disappointment, it was important to just keep going. I think that should be how we live our lives, too. Never spend energy on someone who requires too much attention or pursuit. Go your own way. I regret wasting so much precious time. Life is short, and what was I doing?! Fighting people who didn't share my passion, my vision, my interests? I wonder why I always tried to inspire men in my life to be ambitious, to act, to be geniuses, to build companies, to write books, to be wealthy and giving, instead of being this myself. I was angry for years because I lived with people who were happy with the little things in life. I should not have wasted my time on them!

CHAPTER 22

Russian Doctors

Back to Saint Petersburg. I drew my blood and was waiting for the vaccine. It took around five days. The vaccine was not complete, because we did not have any tumor tissue, but it was better than nothing. Meanwhile, I went to see a young oncologist, Dr. Alkaev, from the Special Academy. Masha's Mom met me near the hospital's reception area in the basement of a two-century old building. The doctor, it turned out, was going to be a little bit late, as he was driving back from a surgery at another location and was stuck in Saint Petersburg traffic. So, Masha's Mom and I decided to explore the hospital grounds.

I followed her through the hallways that smelled of fresh paint and were nicely renovated, through some older buildings that never saw the renovations, and an old dilapidated staircase for staff only. Then, we emerged into an area where it was nice and everything was new. This square compound faced the river Neva and had a huge inner courtyard with the old trees ready to bud. My dad and I came beforehand and were sitting on a garden bench with other patients. I was trying to stay on top of my game and not feel like a patient. In Russia, being a patient means being at the bottom of the Darwinian pyramid. It was ten times worse than in my suburban hospital. Of course, the US suburban hospitals have their own condescensions. I guess it is hard to be human. I have to watch myself all the time or slip into a natural competitive brutality.

I did not expect the doctor to be such a young guy. When we met, I felt immediately that he was the type of person who is just generally good: has a great career, doesn't drink, perhaps is a fantastic father and husband. He was a bit burly and wore the thin rim glasses of a scholar. This time, because I was with the doctor, the staff smiled and greeted us. I knew very well that, if I were there alone, as an outsider, I would be yelled at and pushed around, as a usual "patient:"a weak one who has to suffer and wait.

At first, we were trying to look at my scans on the flash drive that I brought with me, but the Russian computer did not have the right application to open the image files. Dr. Alkaev called up his buddies, somewhere in the guts of the hospital, which I doubt had any IT department. I think these were other young doctors. They quickly installed the program and we were able to look at the scans.

He threw the usual series of questions at me.

"When were you diagnosed?"

"In February."

"When did you have the surgery?"

"A month ago."

"What did they suggest?"

"Chemotherapy.Taxol and cisplatin."

"Okay, good. They know what they are doing."

"What is the primary source?"

"What?"

"Never mind."

We waited, a little, for a guy in the exam room next door to finish. The exam room was very old fashioned with white tiles like in old hospitals that have been rebuilt and remodeled one hundred times. I saw a hospital of that era on Staten Island. We went there with my children's school, and I remember that look of the rooms and equipment: different yet very familiar. In Russia, a lot of things were frozen in the time before art deco, before plastic. There would be bottles made of thick glass, glass test tubes, and steel instruments. Dr. Alkaev made a quick exam and we went out to his office again, to continue our conversation. Then, he thought of something.

"Wait a second," he said. "Let's do an ultrasound."

He quickly pulled out an ultrasound device, an ultramodern, expensive type, very small. I was still sitting in a chair, caught in the middle of a sentence.

"Wait," the doctor said,"What's that?"

"What?"

"Did anyone tell you, you have a liquid in your right lung?"

"No. I believe not."

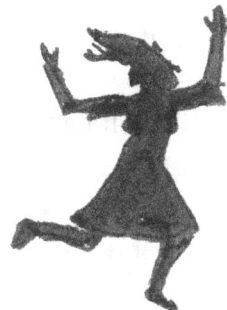

"Are you coughing or having shortness of breath?"

"I was a little bit, right after surgery. They told me it was nothing serious. And maybe I am but, I don't know..."

"You have a lot of liquid. I am surprised you are feeling well."

It's true, I was feeling well. Especially after the immediate chemo effects were gone, I realized that I was feeling very well. I started to breath well. I had a lot of energy.

"How much liquid?" I asked.

"I would say at least a liter. Or to be safe... definitely half a liter."

"Wow. What shall I do now?"

"Well, we definitely need to take it out. It is not a complicated procedure. Would you like to do it here? But then you need to tell your doctor and have him look at it. Of course, it is simple, but it is still a surgery. I am not sure if you feel comfortable doing it here and your doctor having no control over it. No, you know what? I would recommend that you wait. Have the procedure done when you get back to Philadelphia."

"Can it wait?"

"I think it can. Obviously, if you had no idea and you are feeling well."

"Isn't it dangerous to fly?"

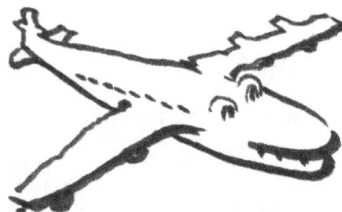

"Well, I guess not. It's half a liter."

"Okay."

"Another thing: this liquid may have cancer cells in it. We'll keep our fingers crossed that it doesn't. "

"Oh no."

"I know. Sorry. "

"What if it does?"

"You know, I think it is better to take it out in Philadelphia. Then, you will do the pathology there, and your doctor will know what to do. They can run the pathology in English. That way they will understand it in America. A Russian pathology report may not be clear for them."

"Okay."

"The only other thing we can do is to do a PET scan on you. I will help you schedule it."

"Okay."

Liquid? With cancer cells in it? This was something unexpected and I almost panicked. I tried not to panic. I did not panic, because I had things to do. I had the vaccine scheduled and then this PET scan, and then I had to go back to Philly in a week for another round of chemotherapy.

I think I had the PET scan the next day. I realized it was a big privilege to do a PET scan. I did not remember what the results were. Somehow, it did not matter anymore. What mattered was that I had to do the dendritic vaccine.

Just to hear another opinion, I went to consult a second doctor, Dr. Kozlova. A friend of mine, Lena, arranged it and we went there together. Lena had just had breast cancer and she knew this hospital. She worked with a different set of doctors, but still she wanted me to go and listen to them. It was an acclaimed Cancer Center in Pesochnaya, outside the city limits. This Pesochnaya Center always had an aura of death; a place no one wanted to know about. We took a metro to the final stop, and then a shuttle bus to Pesochnaya. We came rather early in the morning, and had to wait in line. The receptionists were old Soviet era style monsters, who yelled at us and tried to discipline us in every way. It was a paid visit, meaning entirely out-of-pocket. By American standards, the price was surprisingly inexpensive but, for many Russians, it would have been unaffordable.

At first it was not clear if the doctor would have time to see me or not, but then they decided she would. There were whispers and hints I didn't understand at all. I don't remember if I ended up paying extra, but I felt like a criminal. Was I supposed to be in collusion with the doctor, or against her? The message was very complex and perhaps I did not understand it because it's been so long since I have lived in Russia. When I somehow, either legally or with some winking, made it to the exam room, I was appalled. I had to hold my breath.

There were two or three gynecologic chairs in the room, separated by a screen. Also, separated by a couple of other screens, were women who were waiting for their turn on one of the chairs. I think there were two doctors. Everybody in the room could hear everything that the doctors were discussing with their patients. I climbed up into one of the chairs and the woman doctor made an exam. I heard how she talked with the patient right before me: rude, strong, authoritative. She was there to blame the patient because, obviously, it was all the patient's fault. How could she get so sick?! That attitude was very prevalent in the Soviet era medicine, and I truly hated it. The poor patients accepted the tone and the game of being guilty. I found it unacceptable. I quickly told the intimidating doctor, who was eying me like a police officer, that I actually live in America. The effect was enough to disrupt the role playing, and I did succeed in going through with the exam without being made to feel guilty.

After the exam and telling my story to everyone on the room, I was permitted to enter the office of the doctor I'd come to see. Dr Kozlova was cruel and surreal. She was wearing a fantasy boutique style dress completed with elaborate earrings, necklace, and equally theatrical make up. She was a bird of paradise in the harsh halls of this Cancer Castle. In another world, she might have become a subject of ridicule for lower personnel, but she seemed too powerful to allow any deviation from discipline and respect for hierarchy. She was very colorful in a way a dictator can be. I can only imagine how many struggles she endured to become

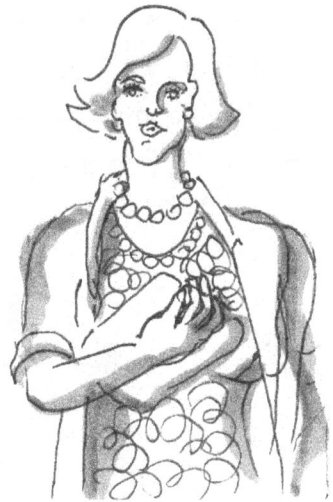

a female doctor, especially one in a position of power. Defined by her battles, she wanted to prove her professional superiority, especially over her American counterparts.

"So, how did you end up like this?" Dr. Kozlova asked me.

I had been trying to avoid exactly this, but I was losing. I was weak and tired, and she knew her game.

"Tell me. What did they do to you there?" She was curious and critical at the same time.

"I had surgery, then I am getting chemo."

"Wrong. In Europe they do chemo first, then surgery, then chemo again."

It sort of made sense, now. I started to suspect that the fluid came into my lungs while I was recovering from surgery, not doing anything to stop cancer. I left feeling guilty for all my sins, my self-confidence destroyed.

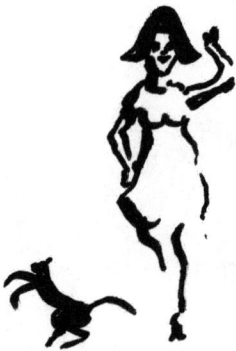

CHAPTER 23

My Dendritic Vaccine

By the end of the week it was time for my dendritic cell vaccination. It would be only half of the vaccine, because the full one would ideally include an antigen of tumor tissue. Still, the vaccine would boost my immune system which was worn out and confused by cancer.

> I <

When I was diagnosed, I had no idea what a dendritic vaccine was. I vaguely remembered, from an immunology class, that dendritic cells were one of many types of immune system white cells. A variety of immune system cells work together as an army to recognize and kill enemy cells. Sometimes something doesn't work and the enemy doesn't get killed.

The first step of solving the problem is to determine the stage at which the malfunction occurred. It's similar to the way a programmer would debug software. Was it that T-killer cells did not fire and attack? If so, why didn't they? Did they know who the enemy was? What if they didn't? What could cause that? Was it that T-helper cells did not pass the information to the T-killer, as in the case of AIDS, when T-helpers are infected by a virus and don't do their job? And how do the T-helper cells recognize enemy cells?

Our investigation starts by determining whether or not dendritic cells are passing along the signals they are supposed to. Dendritic cells pass on signals by digesting the proteins they encounter. Tumor cells shed all kinds of proteins, good and bad. A protein is like a bag of balls, and the dendritic cell chops the bag into its individual balls (epitopes), and then presents them on its surface receptor for the other immune system cells as descriptions of enemy cells. It says, "Everybody who is carrying this red ball with stripes is on Team Cancer." The baseball glove-like pockets that hold the enemy protein are called MHC2.

The next link in the communication chain is the T-helper (or T-regulatory) cell. He sees the glove and the red ball with the stripes in it that the dendritic cell presents. The T-helper has to think. He does not know if all the guys with the red balls with stripes are bad guys. What if some normal cells have the same protein in them and are carrying them on their surface? T-helper has to go back somewhere and ask the question: Do we know if any of our own has the same signature ball in its MHC pocket?

If no, the T-helper cell gives the go signal to the T-killer cell. This T-killer warrior cell, who has seen and recognized the red ball with the stripes, quickly divides to form a million member army. They surround enemy cells doing a flirty dance. They pretend to be loving toward the suspect cells until they are close enough to identify them, conclusively. When they've isolated and identified an enemy cell, the T-killer cells attack it with dagger-like appendages, inject deadly poison, and watch as the enemy disintegrates.

In a lab, we can provide dendritic cells (the spies in the field) with samples of cancerous tissue which they will then present an accurate image of. Then we facilitate the meeting of these dendritic cells with T-helpers (our decision-making officers) and T-killers (the order-executing soldiers). We can do all this on a lab bench and then inject our patient with immune cells that will attack cancerous cells.

ᴘ II ᴄ

We know that cells speak a language of receptor affinity: to the receptors on the surface of other cells and to signal molecules. When a T-killer cell has affinity to receptor MHC ("a glove") with a short portion of a "bad" protein ("a ball") on the surface of a cancer cell, these cells "kiss." For example, Dr. Carl June from UPenn created the super sticky T-cell by genetically engineering the "perfect" receptor to recognize cancer antigen. The T-cell – B-cell chimeric antigen receptor (CAR) would stick to a cancer antigen stronger than the natural T-cell receptor. It is great, but not always. Perhaps because there are other, yet unknown, players, signaling to each other via yet unknown signals to stop the attack. Or never launch.

Would cracking that language mean that we could correct the dialogue between a cancer cell and the immune system? Can we, in our human language, fathom the multi-layered nature of a beast who pretends to be one of our own but is in fact an enemy? The qualities of a cancer cell are just as evasive as the metaphors that keep running away from me. You can ask ten immunologists and they will all draw different pictures with different words. Certain immune system cells can take on any role, for instance, where others may be capable only of performing certain tasks. Scientists learn new things about immune system functions every day.

One day, we may completely describe the immune system and how it reacts on cancer in every case. Still the system is so called "complex" – as weather – something me and my father would have conversations about when I was a school-girl. With every advance in details, we can hope to find that magic combination of events that need to happen to trigger the immune system to target cancer.

"There is something else," Dr. Dmitry told us, when we saw him for the first time. "I am shutting down the immune suppression genes. Let me know if this is okay with you."

We had no idea what he was asking. Dr. Dmitry explained in a little more detail.

"There are cases when the vaccine does not work, and I think this is because there are strong immune suppression mechanisms. So, I am trying to stop the chain of signals associated with the suppressor genes. Like the cells don't react to the suppression because they have no receptors."

We thought about it.

"You don't have to give the answer now."

"Oh no, no. We are fine. Ready."

My father was not ignorant about immunology anymore. He bought a book for us, and was studying it on his own. Now was his chance to give back to humanity in a way – now, when his daughter's life was dependent on his ability to think within the "complex" situation.

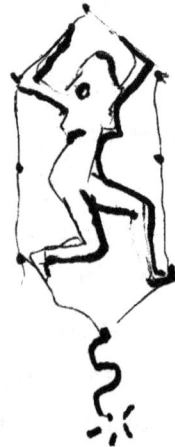

"So, basically what is happening is that there could be a non-specific immune response?"

"Hmm." He was right. He did his reading. He understood a lot of things about the immune system now.

He continued to think out loud: "And it is akin to an auto-immune something..."

"Hmm..." Wow, I thought. He got that. He IS a genius. While I was with my friend at all these fabulous Saint Petersburg concerts he swallowed the whole immunology book. Because he was exactly right: if you suppress the mechanism of suppression, you unsuppress the killing T-cells (if this is how it works). But then I recalled that Natasha, his second wife, had an autoimmune disease and that he, being who he is, a person who believes nobody and is capable of having courage and perseverance to venture into any book and any field of knowledge, studied this for her in depth. So he was not totally naïve to the notions of immunology.

"So the worst thing that can happen is an auto-immune something..."

"But, you say other people are tolerating it well..."

"Yes."

"Good, then. We have no problem with that."

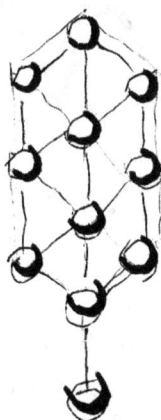

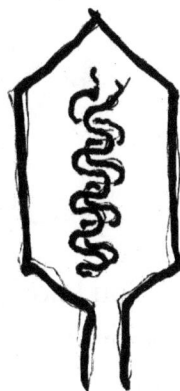

"Finally," I said, "it is your chance to use your brain power for something that we really need! Isn't it nice?"

"Perhaps," he grunted. But I think he had stopped reading when I started to feel better and no longer seemed in immediate danger.

One day, my vaccine was ready. I was sure that the vaccine was the ultimate answer. I had no doubt it would work. This certitude was stirred in me by the honest, stubborn, faith and knowledge of Dr. Petrov. They kept telling me that, if Dr. Petrov was cured, I would be, too. Vika also deeply and blindly believed that Dr. Dmitry was a miracle worker. I gave in to this hope, gladly. It was so firm and all-encompassing. I just knew that the vaccine would have miraculous results. This assuredness calmed me and I was suddenly very capable of dealing with all the messes in my life. It was like a path.

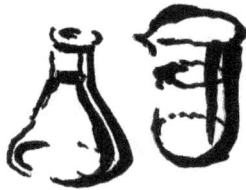

☙ III ❧

"You know what," Dr. Dmitry said once in passing, "You should buy some prednisolone in case you have too strong of a reaction. It rarely happens except with post-surgical patients, who are very prone to a strong immune reaction. It happened with Dr. Petrov. I saw him right after his surgery. He had a very strong reaction."

I knew the story from the Petrovs.

"Anya, you have to weigh the risks. We knew, because we knew as scientists, that Dr. Petrov's chances were zero. We had to vaccinate, before it was too late."

I heard this story enough times to remember every word.

"So what if he suffered somewhat from a little shock? We dealt with it. Too bad there was no solution without risks, but we knew he would have died very quickly if he did not have the dendritic vaccine. We saved him. As you know."

My father was much more frightened than I was. We hired a taxi to Dr. Dmitry's with the instructions to wait for us outside. The injection and the little discussion took about twenty minutes. After the injection, I took prednisolone and we took the taxi home. It was not a real taxi. It was an old Lada and a Tajik driver we hired to drive us around. I think his real name was Mahmud but he called himself Alex, a totally American name in Saint Petersburg. When we were inside, he would wait and doze off, listening to music in his car. Riding home through the night, in the old rusty Lada, we waited for signs of an immune attack. I started to have a fever while we were still in the car and some shaking that I tried to hide.

Whenever he paid the driver, my father thought it was funny to pretend not to have any money. It was always a ritual: he would ask the driver to turn the light on. Then he would start looking for his wallet in the depths of his worn out bag. Then he would look at his wallet with suspicion. Then he would get the bill out from the wallet, stretch out his arm and with a grin and give the bill to the driver, with a nice tip. Even though he knew the routine, the driver would worry, every time, and snatch the bill from my father's fingers. I remember waiting in the car for this endless charade to be over so I could go inside.

At home, we sat down to have some tea.

"How are you feeling? Any fever?"

"Look, she is shaking..." My father pointed at me.

I was shaking, it was true. I couldn't deny it, anymore.

My father touched my forehead with his palm, trying to get an idea if I also had a high temperature.

"Do you have a fever, too?"

"I don't know."

We had some tea.

"Are you shaking?"

We were sitting at the kitchen table and having tea.

"Are you shaking?"

At some point, the shaking was almost gone. I don't remember when, maybe when I went to take a hot shower. I think I took another prednisolone. Then, I went to bed and that was it. The dendritic cells started their cleansing, swooping, action in my body.

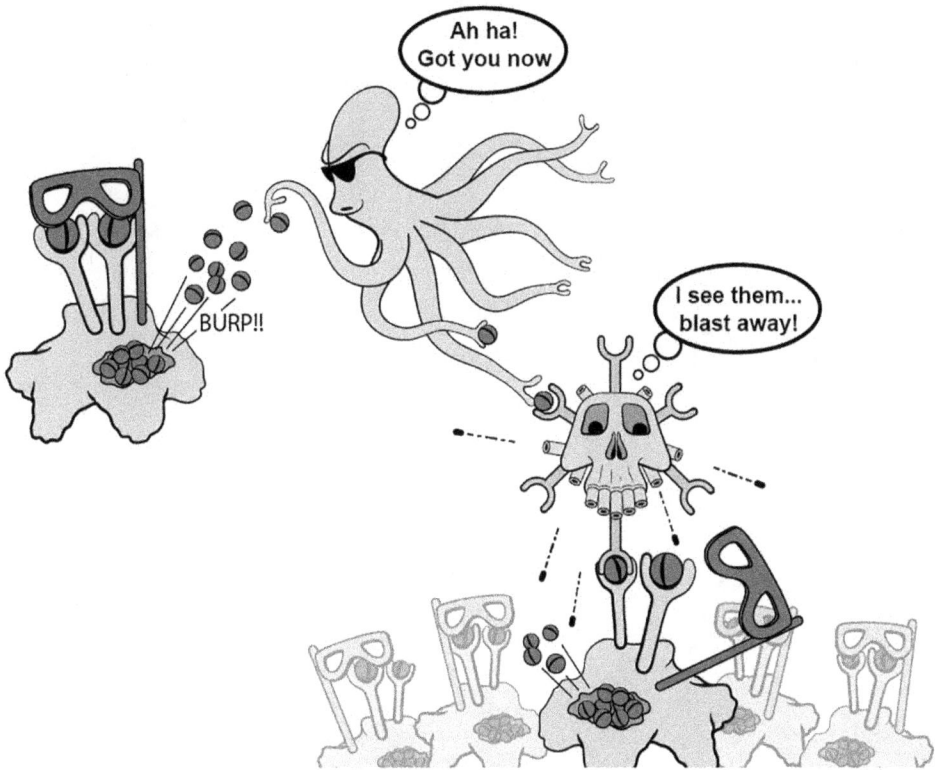

CHAPTER 24
Louise Hay

When I got sick, a friend recommended the book *Heal Your Life* by Louise Hay. It is the story of a woman who transformed herself through positive thinking. She survived cancer and became a contented, healthy, beautiful person in harmony with the world and herself.

Perhaps a day walk under the winter sun, breathing cold fresh air and appreciating it consciously, falling asleep during a slow Sunday afternoon, riding a bike, trembling, holding a yoga pose is happiness. I read about it before I got sick, and it seemed the most boring and least relevant combination of words, fake and unsubstantiated. Now, I see I was killing myself with negative thinking. Most of all, I made myself vulnerable to cancer by living the way I did: overly critical of myself, overly critical of others, demanding that the world conform to my unrealistic expectations.

I read it in the memoirs of those who had cancer: they say the time of the fight was one of the best in their lives. I can attest to this notion. For me, it was the realization that my death would cause so much sadness. My family, my friends, my colleagues, people I never met. They all cared. I had no idea how beautiful my life was, how many true friends I really had.

Before this realization, I never really enjoyed life. There was always something I was missing, something not done right, not started, not finished. I promised my father I would become a great scientist. I had many accomplishments he was proud of, such as becoming a wife and mother, but I was so busy obsessing about the goals I hadn't achieved, such as mastering German. I never let myself really live.

Suddenly, I felt light and happy. All my worries fell away. I felt free. I was happy all the time. Driving to appointments, listening to music, I felt better than ever before. Should I bother about the leaking roof if I am about to die? I decided my husband would be able to take care of it. I had thoughts like: Please let me live to wear the boots I bought in Paris! All that mattered was time. I did worry about my children's futures, but that was the only thing I was worried about.

I would like to take a moment to share some of my favorite Louise Hay quotes:

> *Then one day I was diagnosed with cancer.*
> *With my background of being raped at five and*
> *having been a battered child, it was no wonder I*
> *manifested cancer in the Vaginal area.*
>
> *If I had an operation to get rid of the cancer and*
> *didn't clear the mental pattern that created it,*
> *then the doctors would just keep cutting Louise*
> *until there was no more Louise to cut. I didn't*
> *like that idea.*
>
> *If I had the operation to remove the cancerous*
> *growth and also cleared the mental pattern*
> *that was causing the cancer, then it wouldn't*
> *return. If cancer or any other illness returns,*
> *I don't believe that it's because they didn't "get*

it all out," but rather that the patient has made no mental change. He or she just re-creates the same illness, perhaps in a different part of the body.

I also believed that if I could clear the mental pattern that created this cancer, then I wouldn't even need the operation. So I bargained for time, and the doctors grudgingly gave me three months when I said I didn't have the money.

Being starved for love and affection and possessing virtually no self-worth, I willingly gave my body to whoever was kind to me; and just after my 16th birthday, I gave birth to a baby girl.

I knew that cancer was a dis-ease of deep resentment that has been held for a long time until it literally eats away at the body. I had been refusing to be willing to dissolve all the anger and resentment at "them" over my childhood. There was no time to waste; I had a lot of work to do… I knew I had to clear the patterns of resentment that I'd been holding since childhood. It was imperative for me to let go of the blame. (Hay 11)

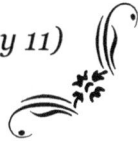

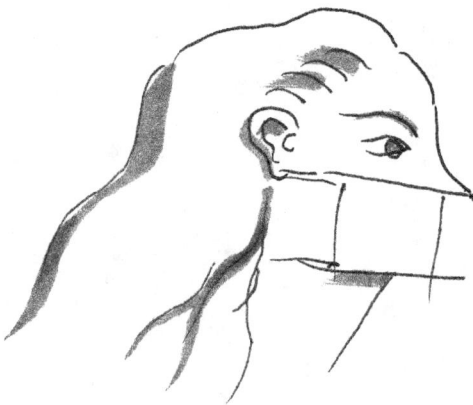

CHAPTER 25

The Little Things

When I came to Saint Petersburg for the first time, after the first chemo, I stayed with my father and Natasha, his second wife, while my mother stayed behind in the US, taking care of my children. I had appointments all over the city every day, and had to avoid taking the metro with its crowds, out of fear of infection. Saint Petersburg flu was something I could not afford at that time. After chemo, I was warned by my American doctors that I would be prone to infections because my immune system would be weakened. I sometimes wore a mask on the plane, which caused some surprised glances. I was dedicated to wearing it, even though I dreaded looking weird. *Never mind*, I thought, I *can bear your stupid stares.*

For some reason, I don't remember now, instead of a taxi we started to hire drivers in old Soviet Lada cars. They were cheap, punctual, and polite. We found them near our building one day. They were all members of one family of endless number of cousins and brothers from Tajikistan who moved to Saint Petersburg for work and opportunity. We rode in one of these decrepit cars, with questionable seat belts and Tajik music set on loud. Through the city of grand imperial palaces and centennial snobs, we sat in the backs of these little rusty Ladas, like ghosts. The driver's stories were about his wife and daughter who stayed behind in Tajikistan, but all these men were here to make a living, send money back, and live happily ever after. The guy suggested he would give us a discount if we would hire him on a regular basis, and so we did. So, now, we were riding in an old Lada through Saint Petersburg all the time, recklessly cutting corners and trying to make it before the red lights. I thought to myself that it wouldn't be so bad to die in a car accident, given that I was already dying of cancer. But, I always buckled myself in, just in case.

Again, I would think of the irony of all my previous attempts to be safe. I guess it's like soldiers in war. You may be about to die; should you bother brushing your teeth? I actually know several people who stopped brushing their teeth because they were soldiers battling away at their invisible wars with cancer, or the world of political oppression by the KGB (in the olden days), or so many other kinds of private wars. Then, when the war was over, they had dental problems. They won but they did not look like it. That is part of why I decided to continue bothering about all the little things.

Also, at this time, I learned to love myself. I guess self-love can come in so many different ways. In my case, it came through my friendships. I realized how much so many people would miss me that I couldn't help but love myself through my love for them. I learned not to worry about my guilts and imperfections, my inability to reach my own goals, and I stopped all the self-punishment I'd been loading on myself for no reason. One of my goals was to learn German. I had tried for many years but I still hadn't mastered the wonderful language of Goethe and Freud. It was something I'd felt bad about since I was fourteen. I wanted to be as great as my father, who spoke German fluently. From time to time during his intellectual instructions, he would mention that he read Schopenhauer in the original. That would make me pale in the face. He seemed such a cultured giant and I longed to learn everything that made him that way, especially the German language.

I studied English pretty well, but that did not help with Schopenhauer. My father also liked to brag how he, as a young boy, lived in Berlin after the war. He bragged about how he went to a German school, how my grandfather had a company car and a driver, and a big German house, food and money, how he liked to chat with the driver, and how my grandma used to help the family of the the driver's family. I would sit tight. I was impressed hearing all his German stories. This Germany was part of me through my father, a metaphor of heroic deeds and intellectual super ego. These were the childhood stories I loved and hated.

My father often spoke to impress and to shine in the sequins of his beautiful boyish princehood. We often talked, late at night, sitting in our kitchen on the 4th floor of an ugly cinder block apartment for Soviet workers. His intellectual iridescence worked on me. I adored the unachievable father in me.

It was still working until my brutal awakening that spring of 2009. Suddenly, German did not matter anymore. This glittering chandelier of my father's intellectual achievements loomed above me when I was a little child at the kitchen table. Only when I was afraid for my life, only then did I find myself in a free space. Only then did I understand its crushing weight. That was very liberating. No more German.

After a while the relief faded, I am occasionally feeling guilty that I did not bother to learn something (only this time it's French), but I remember the liberation moment well. Sometimes I try to connect back to that feeling. Now, I am lucky to have a therapist who helps deal with my German chandelier when it acutely reappears. Then it fades again.

**DEDICATION &
CERTIFICATION OF
THANKS TO:**

*Anna, Michael
and Sasha
Gutkin*

**ANNA THANKS YOU FOR
YOUR KIND SUPPORT!**

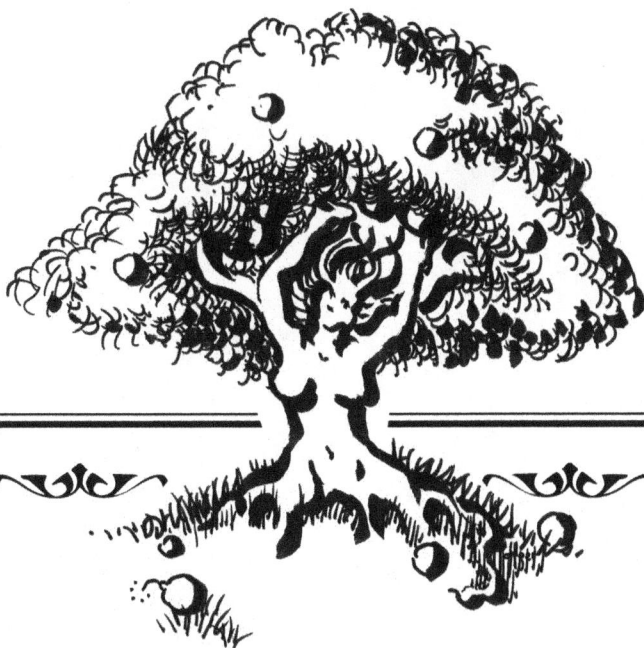

CHAPTER 26

No Problem

I flew back to Philly and immediately called Dr. Mayor, the surgeon who had done my surgery. I announced breaking news: I had fluid in my lungs.

"Liquid? Pleural effusion? I don't deal with lungs. Call Dr. Mendax and she... I am sure she will take care of it."

"What?"

"My territory is below the waist line."

I was devastated, again. The doctor I'd hoped would be my primary physician was disappearing right before my eyes. I disliked Dr. Mendax, the oncologist the surgeon had recommended. She always looked me in the eye with a trained expression of commiseration. She did this when I told her about the fluid in my lungs.

"Oh well. Chemo should take care of the fluid, even if it is malignant," she said.

"Do you think it is malignant?"

"I am pretty sure."

"Ogh!"

"But you should not worry too much because the next chemo should take care of it." Chemo was the only solution Dr. Mendax ever recommended.

"Are you sure?" I asked, just for fun. She had looked me in the eye when she had confidently lied about the clinical trials before.

"Of course."

Of course.

"But you know what," she looked thoughtful for a while and then overconfident again. "Let's make you an appointment with the pulmonologist. He is a wonderful man."

"And what is it for?"

"He will drain the liquid and we will make a pathology test for malignancy. In the meanwhile let's do your chemo. You are already scheduled, right?"

I sat for another chemotherapy treatment, then. I was already so skeptical about this woman and about this place in general. That day, in that room where everybody was sitting in their recliners with IV drippers connecting to their ports or open veins, a woman told me that Dr. Mendax had not noticed a new growth of cancer until it was rather late. "Did not notice! Explain me how that could be!" This poor woman was very upset about her ordeal and how Dr. Mendax kept saying, "It's all right," when the situation was dire and dangerous. I shared my liquid in the lungs story. We both realized we were at the wrong place.

"They will keep saying 'it's all right,' until you die," she said. "They keep saying 'sorry,' and 'that's all right,' and they lie." Chemo took about three hours. By the end, I realized I had to look for a new doctor.

CHAPTER 27

Integrative Medicine

I was in a constant shuffle of appointments, travel, tickets, logistics, blood tests, vaccines, listening to advice, reading, making calls to make appointments that came from the advice, driving to appointments, driving from appointments, driving to the airport, hanging out at the airports in my mask.

I was, in the rare moments when I was not doing all these mandatory things, reading online about immunotherapy. I did a search on "immunotherapy and Philadelphia" and found a paper by a Dr. Chaikin, who was referenced as working at UPenn. I sent the paper to Dr. Dmitry. "Yes, that's it, very good," Dr. Dmitry replied. "They are using an antibody to CTL4 to shut down immunosuppression." All this meant nothing to me at that point. It would take me around three more years to appreciate what Dr. Dmitry was saying, but the acknowledgment of Dr. Chaikin's work was everything I needed at the time.

I wrote an email, immediately. The next thing I knew, I had made an appointment! We exchanged another couple of usual emails where I arranged to send him all the X-rays and paper work I had accumulated going to my million and four doctors.

One email apologized for the lack of a gruesome colonoscopy. This had been such a sticking point with my very first and very insistent doctor. He demanded I do a painful colonoscopy test while I was barely walking, bleeding and weak. He also threatened that he would not perform my surgery if I did not have this done, and called me several times. When I told him I had found another doctor, he became so mad he yelled at me on the phone trying to squeeze the name of the doctor out of me. My first doctor had made me feel like a crazy woman in the attic: a subject of justified yelling, an inadequate loser, a retard, guilty of my ailments and stupidity, dependent and afraid of being abandoned by a beautiful, healthy, smart, and totally superior Doctor with a capital D. I felt especially incomplete and imperfect without the colonoscopy. The tone of my emails was fearful and trembling as I asked if I was worthy to see Dr. Chaikin without the colonoscopy test.

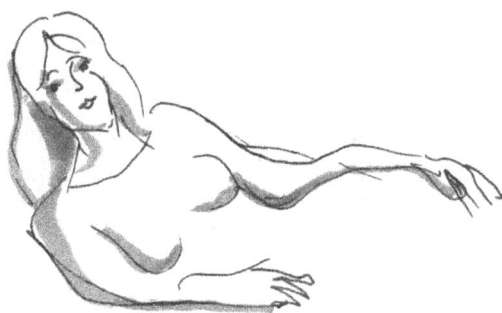

"Why would you need one?" he replied, "not routine."

I was very happy. *Finally!* I thought, *I am in really good hands!* And I was.

I went to UPenn soon to see Dr. Chaikin. What a different institution it was compared to all other hospitals I had visited! It made a psychological difference right from the get-go, right from the receptionist in the Abramson Cancer Center. This hospital was an architectural masterpiece with a high dome of glass and steel above a huge open public space filled with a buzz of conversations and coffee machines, sounds of steps, elevators going up and down in glass casings making nurses and doctors look tiny under five stories of air below the open sky. The receptionists would give you all their attention; they would care for you and make sure you found your directions in this airy and fantastic palace of health.

Yet another receptionist at the office of gynecologic oncology was very helpful. She was also very casual and accessible, and she managed to make me feel like her best friend. She would complement my wigs, my makeup, my shoes, and she did it with such a natural interest that I forgot she was doing it for money. She was very genuine. She would tell me stories about herself too. What a joy after so many battles with receptionists! She later left to do her MBA, but the man who replaced her was as kind and helpful as she was. They all were. It was heavenly. I sighed with relief.

Dr. Chaikin told me we would have to start me on a new chemical. "You are young," he said, "and can do an aggressive protocol." I began two different types of chemotherapy session, repeated every month, for eight months. One would be three hours and would include intravenous taxol. Then, in three weeks, I would need to spend a night at the hospital where they would do a slow intravenous injection of carboplatinum and also, through a port, another drug would be delivered inside my belly. The port needed to be surgically installed, and they would take it out after the chemo completed in eight to ten months. I said yes to everything and made an appointment for the port surgery.

Then we had to address the *pleural effusion*. Dr. Chaikin quickly called someone in Pulmonology.

"What's pleurodesis?"

"It is a procedure. ...where...talc...layers... adhesion... drained through a tubing that is connected to a container."

"What??"

An image of a container attached to my lungs made me cringe. I already had an attached container before, when I was recovering from the surgery, I did not mind it before, but I had just gotten rid of it and was against any other auxiliary device that could be attached to me. It just did not sound right. And the whole talc treatment sounded very pessimistic, very "last options before you die peacefully." Before I could collect my thoughts into a definite opinion, he continued:

"I've got you an appointment with a pulmonologist. He is good. He will have a look and he will remove the liquid. Maybe we will need pleurodesis. It's a tube that is perma- nently attached to your lungs to drain the new liquid."

It was going great. I did not have to be attached and talced immediately. I sighed with relief and gently pushed my agenda.

"I will need the liquid for myself," I said.

"Not possible. The liquid belongs to the University. It's a policy."

That was a bomb. I needed this liquid for my vaccine, as
we agreed with Dr. Dmitry. It was yet another time out of
many times when I was shocked and devastated. I begged a
little more, but he was stern. The University would not give
me the liquid from my own lung. I don't remember what
I told him about why I needed the liquid. I could not tell
him of course that I was doing an immunotherapy vaccine
in Russia. I was not sure, myself, what could happen if I
combined all those therapies. It even bothered me that I
would not be able to tell what had worked and what hadn't.
I don't know why! Perhaps our minds are trained to isolate
causes: one and only one remedy. Only much later did I
start to realize how restrictive this thought pattern was. I
understand, now, there are many ways in which we can help
our body and we should not eliminate any one of them for
the sake of knowing decisively which one did the trick.

I shared with Dr. Dmitry my discomfort of not knowing
which therapy would really work if I tried many remedies,
all at the same time. At some point, I mumbled something
about me using other treatments to boost my immune
system and Dr. Chaikin said that would be a good thing,
perhaps. He did not ask what it was and I didn't tell him
about the dendritic vaccines. His answer cured me from
the deep subconscious fear of breaking the logic that was
ruling my life. "Why would you care what exactly cures
you?" he said. This phrase stuck in mind, since then,
and I repeat it to others. I have, since, seen many people
who, without knowing, felt the need to limit themselves
to a single treatment, letting go all other things including
possible cures. Our body needs help from many directions.
A collective effort can multiply results in the same way that

one man is not enough to push a stalled car off the road, but three can succeed.

My next destination was the office of Integrative Medicine. The doctor was kind and understanding. I felt I'd been given permission to do everything I could. I realized that, in the office of the doctor with two thousand years of Jewish compassion pouring through his eyes, I could talk about my many approaches without fear.

Conventional doctors, I think, are still governed by the premise of a single treatment. If I presented them with something they did not know, they would panic visibly. It was fear of approving a combination that might have unknown side effects. They would have told me to stop all additional treatments, in fear of responsibility. Doctors' fear of litigation is something I had to think about and protect them from. I always gave them only partial information and instinctively did not share anything with a doctor that was outside his realm of everyday practice. I did not want to make my good doctors uncomfortable, even though, I must admit, I enjoyed teasing the bad, pompous ones. However every good doctor wanted me to survive. They understood that it was my battle, and I was encouraged to save myself any way I could find.

CHAPTER 28

Operation Antigen

❮ I ❯

I was still scheduled for chemotherapy with the The Highly Recommended But Lying Dr. Mendax. I didn't want to let her know I was leaving before I already had. I started to master the art of light-hearted evasions, semi-truths, running the bases while the ball of my options was in the air. I had to learn how to quickly recover from the devastation of having been tricked out of clinical trials with lies. I had to keep running.

I was being less than honest with Dr. Chaikin, too. When he said it would be impossible for me to keep any of the fluid removed from my lungs at UPenn, I had no choice but to explore other options. I wound up going back to an earlier hospital, carrying a big backpack stuffed with all my X-rays, reports, folders, and all the papers I had accumulated in my journey so far. I think I looked pretty miserable when I appeared at the office of this secret pulmonologist, Dr. Scheinberg. He was exactly the type of smart, kind, and calm doctor whose calm and listening strengthens you. He looked at me with awe when I told him about my travails: about going to Russia and discovering the fluid in my lungs there. I hid my emotions about the care I had received, or rather had not received, at his hospital. How was it possible that I had to go to Russia (to Russia!) to find out I had half a liter of liquid in my lungs? He complimented my courage.

Dr. Scheinberg said he didn't mind if I took some of the fluid with me! Thank you, God! It was just the break in the clouds I needed and things started to look better again. I thanked the Universe for this kind pulmonologist. Because of people like him, I am optimistic about humanity. In my mind, he exemplified that quality in certain people that makes them willing to risk themselves for the sake of others, unabashed in their stern humanity. I was so tired of running from place to rejecting place: tired and worn out by the unforgiving system.

⊀ II ⊁

We knew we would have the fluid at twelve o'clock on a Friday. That moment, the antigen's clock would begin to tick. How would we get it to Russia? I was tired from the recent flight and I had the surgery and the chemo ahead of me, too. We knew the life of the fluid was 24-48 hours. Within this time, it had to be on the bench of the lab in Russia. We also had to find someone who worked with tissue cultures because the cells had to be shipped in a certain medium for growing tissue cultures and these flasks would have to be prepared in a specific way. We asked many friends and, through one friend, we found someone with the necessary skills and materials. He found my story compelling and decided to help. When I came to his house to pick up the prepared flasks, his wife opened the door. "What? Anya?!" It happened that we knew each other! She had no idea whom the flasks were for. When I told her my story, she was so sincerely saddened that I think she felt worse than I did. My story brought us much closer together and, if not for the help of her husband, who I never met, I might not have gotten my vaccine in time.

Armed with the flasks hidden in my backpack, I marched to the appointment. Dr. Scheinberg took us into a procedure room, a typical room with a curtain, a bed, and a couple of chairs. He was very experienced. Carefully, after tapping my chest for the puncture place, he stuck a needle into my lung. The waters rushed out into a big, old fashioned glass bottle with a rubber stopper. It looked like something from a Russian hospital, so antiquated it was. The first bottle was filled and the doctor changed it for the second. Gosha was sitting there with his eyes wide open. I guess the spectacle of a waters gushing from his wife's lungs was mesmerizing. Then came the third bottle. This was sort of unexpected. Dr. Scheinberg left to get another. The waters continued to leak. When water stopped, there were 4.5 liters altogether. He disconnected the needle, wiped my skin with an alcohol wipe, and left the room so that we could have some privacy with my 4.5 liters of fluid and the flasks. Gosha and I quickly transferred the fluid to the flasks, as much as we could, using a lighter to sterilize the area where we were holding the flasks and the bottles. My microbiology training came in handy, here. When we were done, the doctor came back in. He still had a huge amount of liquid left to do pathology tests. I was ready to kiss him. He was clearly saying to me, by the way he handled the situation, that the only thing he cared about was my life. I will always remember his kind love. This wonderful Dr. Scheinberg was yet another instrumental person in preparing my vaccine. I wish him and his family long years of peace and love.

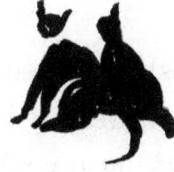

⊀ III ⊁

Gosha grabbed the flasks and rushed to the airport. We knew we only had 48 hours to get the flasks to the lab. Lacking any other option, we decided to ask Russian tourists to carry the liquid to Russia. Gosha rushed from person to person, asking them to take the flasks and carry them in their luggage. They all said, "No."

We'd already used up four precious hours. Someone had to fly to Russia today or tomorrow, or else the cells would die and we'd miss our chance. I considered doing it myself. On a hunch, I called Kira, an old friend of mine from my Saint Petersburg high school. She was an active member in the Russian community of New York. She did not know anyone who was flying to Russia tomorrow, but she knew someone who would if we bought him a ticket. Gosha called Ivan Mikhalych right away. Yes, he would love to visit his family in Moscow for free. Ivan Mikhalych flew the next day.

I was worried that something would happen and that airport security would interfere with Ivan Mikhalych and not let him carry the liquid, so we thought of a back-up plan. We decided to divide the liquid into two parts: we'd send one to Russia for Dr. Dmitry to work on and keep the second part separately, just in case. This back-up liquid, we sent immediately to David Vausse, a cell tissue biologist—a lucky friend for me to have!—who could grow any cells from any source in vitro. Now, we had two batches of my possibly cancerous cells from the suspicious 4.5 liters of liquid in my lungs.

The next morning, Ivan Mikhalych met us at the airport and packed my cells into his luggage. It was already 30 hours since the liquid was taken. My father met Ivan Mikhalych at the airport with the taxi and delivered my fluid to Dr. Dmitry almost 48 hours after the liquid was taken out of my body. Now my cells were in Russia waiting for me to come to Saint Petersburg for the next vaccine round.

CHAPTER 29

Stage Four

The pathology analysis of the liquid from my lungs showed
that it had malignant cells. I read the pathology report in
a flash, unable to concentrate on any other information
but the word "malignant." It was scattered throughout:
malignant... malignancy... malignant...

My body tensed in panic. This news meant that my cancer
had progressed from stage three to stage four, with malignant cells outside of the primary tumor site. The thought of
this news makes me cringe even now. At the same time, if
there had not been malignant cells, Dr. Dmitry would have
not been able to include an antigen in his dendritic vaccine.
These malignant cells could be my salvation. I had expected
this, maybe even hoped for it. I calmed down, choosing
to ignore the gruesome details and focus on my dendritic
vaccine and any other new options I could find. I returned
to Dr. Chaikin, but without the liquid in my lungs.

·· I ··

My first appointment was with Dr. Connolly the bright,
young pulmonologist Dr. Chaikin had praised so highly. He
had a hand-held ultra sound device that he said belonged
to him, personally. This meant I didn't even have to make
another appointment! But, as the two doctors discussed the
ultrasound, my good mood clouded over. Dr. Chaikin mentioned something about "pleurodesis." I heard the words

"talc," "drainage," "tubes," and "on a permanent basis." It sounded like a set of radical and dangerous measures.

The bright, young Dr. Connolly turned to me.

"You look quite strong, carrying this backpack around..."

"I don't want to do it, yet. Can we wait?" I interrupted.

Dr. Connolly put away his ultrasound device and we all looked at the picture of my lungs on the screen. He tried to show me where the right lung looked different from the left lung, and where various organs were. They remained indistinguishable to me in this blurred movie of pulsating inner fleshes and iridescent liquids.

The doctor now prepared to remove the fluid from my lung and save it for Dr. Chaikin's vaccine, puncturing my chest with a needle and draining the liquid into a bottle. This time it was hardly half a liter. "Let me call Dr. Chaikin's *mendicants* to collect this stuff," Dr. Connolly suggested. I was surprised to hear such a rare word and looked at him with interest. "I was an English major in college," he said with a slightly apologetic grin." I was thinking of becoming a writer too," I said. It was a hard truth to admit because, even though I was always writing something, there was never a finished piece. The *mendicants* took a long time to appear, but Dr. Connolly and I sat comfortably together in quiet kinship.

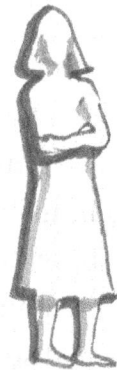

·· II ··

Patients in the lung department are recognized by either of two things: transparent tubes coming out of their nostrils or oxygen tanks that roll by their side. Patients with oxygen tanks ordering pizza at a cafeteria became a normal, even reassuring, sight for me. I think this is how Abramson Cancer Center is designed: with the notion that no human condition is bad and that all deserve the right to acknowledgement. Most hospitals I visited found ways to hide those patients outfitted with unappetizing apparatus or whose conditions might otherwise distress visitors from the general public. The Abramson Center employed the most wonderful understanding of this fact: the only way to remove the stigma against the abnormal is to let it be the norm.

This concern is especially important for hospitals, where each case is truly individual and each patient in need of unique treatment. When I was called back to the office, I had a very disappointing conversation with Dr. Chaikin about my vaccine. He told me that, although they would prepare and store antigenic material for me out of the liquid removed from my lung, I would not qualify for an immunotherapy vaccine until I completed front-line therapy.

"But we all know that front line therapy will never work in the end. Right?" I said.

"Yeah. I am sorry. I can't give you the vaccine, yet."

Front line therapy is the standard chemotherapy treatment given to first time cancer patients. It was accepted that this treatment would not kill all malignant cells. Some would lie dormant for a year or two before starting to divide. This recurrence of cancer would be resistant to the front line chemicals. Each successive round of chemotherapy would use a new chemical and leave resistant cells. Eventually, all known chemotherapy drugs would have been exhausted and then the patient would die.

With immunotherapy, however, a vaccination of immune cells will hunt for cancer cells in all body tissues. It would be like administering a constant treatment. Any cancer cells that did succeed in hiding in a dormant state would be weaker, not stronger. Also, the body's immune response would be increased, as opposed to chemotherapy where immune response is actually compromised.

It did not make any sense I could not get my personalized care. Such inferior treatment was not the will of any person, no doctor or group of conspirators, but was imbedded in the system itself, powerful and blind, dangerously running amok, unless humans interfere.

Who could repair such a broken machine? Doctors are too busy in their labs and attending to their patients to become activists for policy change. Patients, especially cancer patients, are so weakened by their disease that it is almost too much for them even to hope to recover. Patients' spouses are overwhelmed by the increase in their respon- sibilities as they must now compensate for the income and childcare no longer provided by their partners. This absurd system seems not to allow doctors to attend to the patients fully. I have great sympathy towards those doctors who still try to do right for their patients, spending their time looking for a narrow solution that is not putting them in danger legally and yet is a step forward in the care for the sick, navigating the waters carefully in between fear and humanity.

On the way from Philadelphia to JFK in New York, down New Jersey Turnpike exit 12, there is a huge and elaborate oil refinery with many metal spheres and pipes. They smoke through their carefully monitored chimneys. I was discussing immunotherapy with the husband of a friend, complaining about all my unsuccessful attempts to get into treatments, as we drove toward the airport.

"Look," he said, "they have built these expensive, elaborate cancer wards. Why do tiny immunotherapy? All it requires is one little scientist with his one little test tube. How would they explain all their equipment?" We continued to drive silently. I never like "they" and cringe at a notion of any conspiracy theory. However, just like a husband of a cancer patient, my friends all came up with this theory at some point in my journey. However, today, in 2013, immuno-therapy departments are springing up in all Big Pharma companies. And why not? This is the technology that works, and they are making adjustments. In the end, the consumer wins, at least in the capitalist economies. However, this treatment is still not available for the masses of consumers. But I am sure it will, especially if more people would know about it, from this book, for instance.

All I can say is that the increasing difficulty of finding personal treatment in American hospitals was making me extremely grateful that Dr. Dmitry was waiting for me in Russia with his vaccine.

CHAPTER 30

The Health Care Castle

In his novel, the Castle, Franz Kafka, depicts a cruel, self-serving institution functioning without any regard to logic or human interest, including the interests of its creators. Outdated, inflexible, ideology driven, able to pretend to serve a reasonable function and capable of controlling the resources and time of innocent citizens, the institution had become a cancer. In my youth, this book helped me survive the absurdity of the Soviet Empire. It is interesting that a wonderfully eloquent writer, Susan Gubar, in her brutal description of her ovarian cancer journey, makes references to another of Kafka's books, The Trial. Maybe Kafka knew more about cancers than he is given credit for: cancers and empires.

Cancer is an absurdity in the language of our body, where our body's goal is to work as a well-functioning whole. A cancer works toward the absurd idea of building yet another body inside of the one it inhabits. It sucks all the resources out of its host and dies itself. Although pretending to serve the whole, cancer actually undermines its integrity, like a parasite, like an oppressive regime that has fooled some social immune system. The Soviet Empire fell because, in its inefficiency, it ran out of resources but, also, because its citizens could not lie to themselves anymore about the real nature of their authorities or the fact of their increasing depletion. Egyptian, Roman, Byzantine Empires fell because the external enemies were stronger than their overly hierarchical internal systems. Unable to organize their alienated citizens against a common enemy, these ancient empires succumbed to immunodeficiency disorders.

My exposure to the absurdities of the Soviet Empire that were appeased by working through it with Kafka's The Castle, made me far more immune to the frustrations that the absurdities of the health care system brought to me, years later, on American soil. My American friends would take much longer to recognize the absurdity and inhumanity of the Health Care Castle. Anyone dealing with a vast, impersonal institution could benefit from a healthy dose of cynicism. But, I wonder if the metaphor could serve us further. We know that all empires fall. Could cancer fall, just like an empire? Could we find its cure through a common language?

Could one intentionally deplete the Cancer Republic of resources such as glucose delivered by blood vessels formed in the vicinity of a tumor? Or, what external enemy could conquer the Cancer Republic with all its metastasizing lies and grifter cells monopolizing resources until all integrity would be finally compromised? I was completely lost inside the absurdity of the Health Care Castle. Its inner workings, inner logic, its pathways for digesting its patients, its fantastic incomprehensible costs, the undergrounds of the insurance companies who were able to pay the unimag- inable costs of both absolutely essential and the absolutely doubtful treatments: these were all of unimaginable proportions and terribly unsettling.

CHAPTER 31
Meditation

Before I got sick, I always worried about everything: misunderstandings, torn self-esteem, money... What a harmful waste of my precious life! I had been healthy and miserable. After I got sick, I had so much more to be miserable about that I had to overcome it. In the midst of my cynical frustration, my friend, Annette, took me to her meditation practice at the Won Institute of Buddhist Studies in a nearby town of Glenside. The meditation teacher, Glenn Wallis, became a powerful and astonishing presence in my life from that moment forward several crucial years toward recovery.

✦ I ✦

I started to attend his meditation class every Monday night at 7pm, whenever I wasn't off traveling to Russia. There was a group who would get together to sit in silence for an hour, then go on a quiet forest walking meditation. The meeting would end with a thought or a poem that Glenn would recite and offer a kind and passionate interpretation of. Then, everybody would contribute to the discussion. The two hour ceremony would end with everyone feeling a little different than before. These meditations became a fundamentally important thing for me. They were instrumental in teaching me to feel calm and powerful. In the silent world of inside your belly where you connect to Nature, where we belong only as simple beasts trying to analyze our existence, and as a result of thinking this way, my condition became just a condition on the spectrum of life's conditions.

Glenn liked me, and his sympathy and sharing intellect added a lot of cheer to my life. He invited other people from his meditation class to participate in helping me with my life and my treatments. It felt fantastic. In Buddhist tradition, the circle of people who sit together and share the moments of silence during meditation is called "sangha." It felt fantastic to belong to Glenn's sangha. They smiled at me and asked me questions about my wellbeing, about my travels and children.

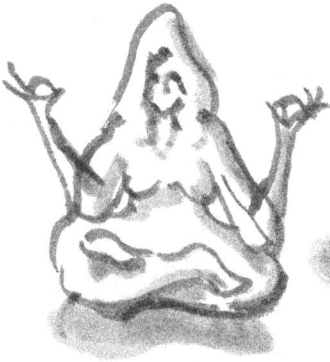

My life was getting better and better. I continued to feel loved by everyone I ever knew. Abandoned connections came alive from my past: colleagues, rivals and enemies made peace with me when they learned about my diagnosis. I realized how much my enemies loved me and this changed my perspective, dramatically. All those people I had mistrusted, not spoken to for years, suddenly started to reach out to me, to cry at my fate, to help in whatever way they could, as if there had never been bad blood between us. I loved feeling those connections again! Seeing so much innate human goodness made me a different person. I had never experienced such clarity. Real life, as I see it now, is just some breaths that you can take, because if you are not breathing there is nothing for you, anyway.

This truth about breathing came to me when I started meditations with Glenn. Breathing while sitting and thinking about breath were the main focus. I realized that my breath was the only connection to my life, not as a path, but as an elemental act of being alive, now. While I breathe, I am here. While we breathe, together, we share air and time. Qualms about lost time—time not spent writing and traveling, time not spent with my children, the various guilts and illusions of daily life—they were all burnt up in the fire of counted breaths.

When I would get to breath number fifty, something would start to happen. I would feel a warm, lightened sensation, full and happy. I came to deeply feel that interconnectedness is a natural way of being. Now, looking back, I see how all those moments of meditation made me what I am today, and I remember this time as one of the most interesting and fruitful in my life. I acquired the ability to question everything. I wondered how, being a scientist, I nevertheless acted on beliefs and superstition rather than on my direct knowledge and facts. So many of my actions were motivated by so many myths: myths inherited from my family, Soviet era societal mythology, American myths, all those myths of all those places to which I belonged at different times. I cannot be sure any time that I act from my truth, but I think I do it much better than before. Breathing and being honest about it had a wonderful effect on me.

✦ II ✦

Glenn has a tremendous ability to feel for others. Perhaps he learned it through years of practice, but I think it's just the way he is. When Annette brought me to his meditation class, I immediately felt surrounded by attention. Every one there took interest in making me feel better. Glen talked to me for hours on end. He listened to me with loving care, trying to understand who I was, trying to help. I was very honest with him, and he knew a lot about my concerns and tribulations.

Money was becoming a bit of an issue for me. I was spending eight hundred to a thousand dollars a month on airplane tickets to fly to Russia. That was a new basic cost of staying alive, like food or shelter. There were, of course, other expenses, too. Glenn asked me about money. "I don't want you to stop any possible treatment because you may be thinking about money," he said. Though I had insurance, and my major doctors were covered, I was going to an acupuncturist a couple times a week and buying a lot of herbal remedies, seeing a naturopathic doctor and taking sodium butyrate. At the end of every meditation, Glenn would announce that "there is a person in need among us and please leave some money to help out." Every Monday night, after every meditation, I would be given money that would make me feel better buying all those endless medicines and going to my acupuncturist – truly not thinking about the costs

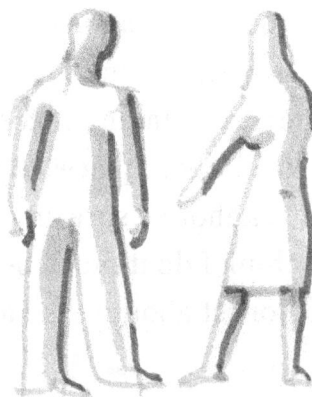

"I don't want you to forgo any treatment for the lack of money," Glenn said. I never felt I could thank Glenn enough for his listening to me, for his accompanying me to the hospital, for being a witness and a mediator. I did thank Glenn many times, but never enough, and never to the full sangha. Writing this ode to my sangha, I realize I owe them a loud and public "Thank you!"

Any time we decide to help someone outside of our immediate family circle, we must weigh whether we can afford the time and resources. Glenn was writing a biography of the Buddha. He must have had to decide the extent to which he would support the writing of his book, an endeavor very important to him, and to what extent he would help me. If the book were a success, it would be a tremendous benefit to his two daughters and to his wife Friederike. Glenn gave of his time freely to help another human being in her time of need, and the other human being was me.

Glenn made a truly a special effort. He was actively engaged in Operation Anna. Mostly, he talked to me. I was in a state of perpetual confusion and often in tears. His listening was reassuring and tranquil. Glenn listened with sympathy and acceptance as I talked about the relationship I had with the world before my illness and the constant struggle for sanity within the Kafkaesque absurdity of the health care system. He listened as I recounted my intellectual history, my secret wishes, my embryonic interest in philosophy

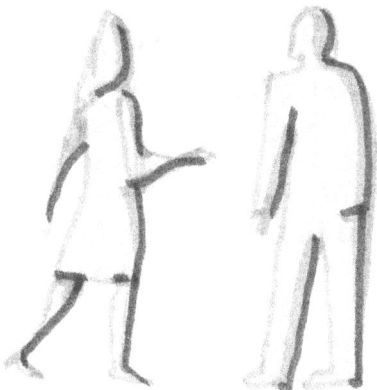

and language that I nursed as a dream, saying: "One day I am going to wake up and write about everything."

Now, after I was helped so tremendously, I look for opportunities to engage in helping others. I know that I can spare the time to listen. Anyone can. It is time taken out from doing our own things, from talking to our own children, from working out at the gym, from writing our own books, from our pleasant routines. I learned the value of time from Glenn, the value of making a decision to spend the precious time of your own life for the sake of another.

Strange, Glenn was not competing with me but was conversing. That was such a rare gift, something I plan to seek for in the future. My pre-cancer life, on the contrary, was filled with fierce competition with Gosha, my boss, my father, the endless questioning of everything I was doing and thus of my worthiness. These calm conversations allowed me to escape the damaging frustration over my Russian family and my jealous boss, to heal and prepare for the long road of treatment that lay ahead.

✦ III ✦

I am breaking a taboo like Susan Gubar knowingly broke when she chose to tell the whole unpleasant truth about her physical suffering, revealing for the first time the ugly details of constipation and diarrhea that a cancer patient goes through, details that were avoided in all the cancer stories.

The taboo I am about to break is to tell the truth of a

different kind of suffering that was part of my cancer journey, the suffering rooted in my long marriage, joyful at the beginning but having become the ground for an uncompromising competition and battles. It took a heavy toll on me. Perhaps it's one of those cases where it's nobody's fault, and the suffering can be stopped if you count your blessings and both leave, instead of staying in the prolonged agony and suffering.

My suffering from those marriage battles was becoming a bomb that was festering inside of me and that blew up in my face as the cancer did one day.

When that happened, Gosha helped me tremendously in my ensuing cancer journey, in fact he was instrumental in getting me where I am today. He handled all the logistics of my travels and some vaccine components, and he stayed with the kids at home taking care of all their needs and the house. I felt free to pursue my health. He gave me this chance and I am very grateful. He loved me. Once he told our common friend Vika: "Money is not a problem. Let's save her no matter what it costs." I wish he told this to me too. At the beginning of illness, my days were filled with frustration and helplessness; he became gentler and stopped competing. I forgot all the battles we had. It clearly did not matter anymore.

As soon as I was getting better, however, we were back to a constant battle of egos, a man in the house against a woman. One might say, he felt threatened, just like any man can be threatened by any woman, they say. I have heard that it's OK, men do it all the time, in self-defense and unknowingly. Perhaps, but these arrows were very hurtful.

I felt that it was taking the toll on my health, and that was very troubling. I felt as if I was in the middle of a never-ending competition. This marriage suffering was as physical as one from constipation or diarrhea. It was as real.

My meditation teacher, a wise and kind woman, suggested to treat my frustration as an ocean wave – just wait till it was over, "because you know it's gonna be over, right?" Right.

When did it start? How did we end up there in this battle?

I thought we started as two equals, equally responsible for each other's happiness and success. We have known each other for so long that we are almost brother and sister. However, with time I realized that he was dealing with expectations that were more "traditional", more "Russian", than mine, with a man as the center of worship, a decision maker, an ultimate authority figure, uncontested and kind by choice. I had a problem with that.

I also had a problem with Gosha's loyalties being with his Russian boys. Their sometimes real, and sometimes perceived judgment became the crucial presence in my family, not the real life that we were living in America. I could just feel these voices whispering their recipes on how to handle my behavior, in my partner's ears. I did not like that, and I wanted to have a partner who would be more present, not just the echo of his peers. Such is the power of tradition that it molds us, but only if we are not conscious about it. Gosha chose the "traditional" model by default; however, I could not accept it and always "rebelled" against our heavy intriguing mix of a traditional marriage exacerbated by our Russian predicament.

I had problem of feeling like I was a "madwoman in the attic" (Susan Gubar thank you for this brilliant metaphor) when I attempted to be myself, to be what I thought I should be in 21ST century America. "Honey, you are crazy" and "Honey, you are inadequate" were so overused in my family. Something so 19th century!

I had a problem with constant competition and battles. I was expecting encouragement and empowerment from my partner. However, we in Russia love battles:that makes it really hard to love inside the Russian tradition. Like everything else, like survival in the cold weather, marriage is a battle that you are supposed to fight. Not a place for love.

20th century Russian History is one of big battles, prosecutions, revenge and punishments. It became the Russian way of life. Stalin's regime punished twenty million people, mostly men, in his concentration camps. Then the Second World War killed another twenty million men. Men became rare and precious. Russian men grow up in an atmosphere of protection and worship, and thus even the best of them drag around their cultural tumor of the mix of privilege, dismissive ignorance towards the rest of the world, and a deep-seeded fear of a regime hunting them down.

This is the power of culture; it is like cancer,deep in all the tissues of our psyche, deeper than skin, deeper than thought. Deeper than love.

CHAPTER 32

The Russian Gender Riddle

Slowly but surely, the disturbing disconnect between men and women in Russia is becoming my signature discussion topic. When I noticed it ten years ago, it was an almost revolutionary observation for me. I stuck to my observation, often ridiculed for being "obsessed" with the topic of Russian men. Time has shown that I noticed something important, that other thoughtful people started to notice as well. Russian women are not happy with Russian men. Of course, there are rare harmonious marriages, always under fierce attack from society with its falling standards for men's behavior. It is an obligation for a Russian man to drink heavily. A patriotic duty. A heroic deed. A tangible way of life.

A typical Russian TV commercial would be a drinking gang of semi-naked beer buddies. The camera would portray them drunk and still drinking. Women rarely appear in commercials at all. Sometimes, an aged woman would advertise cleaning supplies.

Due to many processes, all of them interconnected, Russia has become a society of men. In population genetics terms, Russia was a huge experiment that shifted the population biologically. The main event that occurred was that men became scarce. First the Revolution and the Civil War took millions of men's lives, then Stalin's genocide took twenty million men's lives in the horror of the concentration labor camps and World War II took another twenty million men's lives. Being a devious creature akin to Hitler, Stalin killed the smartest, the bravest, the richest and the best men. This is where the genotype shifted. We are for the most part, offspring of cowards and guards, alas. This, of course, made men rare and prized creatures. That helped lower the standards for men. The society became owned by men and divided into two distinct sub-populations: cowards and guards.

And women.

However, the social myth was not ready for this shift in reality.

Women still expected and wanted traditional things: a man, a marriage, a family, children, a home, a steady routine, education for the kids, security at home. However, men who grew up as prizes had no expectations for themselves, except for just being. It was enough to just be. Just be present. Not only did men die from the cruelties of the regimes; the hatred caused self-inflicted wounds like alcoholism.

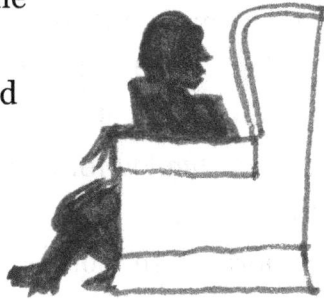

Being alive became an achievement even when a more prosperous and peaceful time came in the 60s. It was a break for the Russian people, and the men started to rebuild their pride. I guess intuitively. It was also the time of the cold war, and the government needed rocket scientists. This was when it started to groom boys into mathematicians, physicists, and engineers. Talented boys were praised and placed into special schools for mathematics.

For families of those boys this was a salvation from the horrors of the damaged society outside the schools.

These boys were destined to go to the Universities and Colleges and be protected from being drafted into the Army as soldiers. These boys from a few big cities were very capable intellectually. They were the cream of the crop men, and they were content for the rest of their lives

With women competing for men, men found it easy not to grow up, not to move beyond that partying roguishness, those drunken selfish jokes. Women were first fighting and then would become deeply disappointed at their spoiled and symbolic male figures. They screamed and yelled in desperation. But why? Everybody was the same. Not just THIS man.

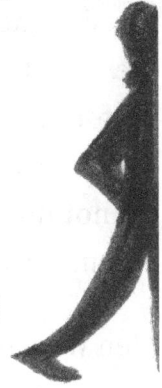

Before the Soviet Union collapse, we lived by a clear and sterile morale where sex was never discussed and almost forbidden. In the nineties, when we suddenly became free to talk about real life, including sex, it became sex only: sex as an obligation, as a cool thing, as a weapon against oppression, a sign of worthiness, suddenly accepted as a propaganda symbol, making machismo a necessary tool in the patriotic toolbox.

It was propped up as the "revolt of the true man." The media included two things that went together ideologically but did not go together physiologically: sex and alcohol. The poor Russian men, who had a load of performance expectations on their shoulders, "had" to be sex machines and, at the same time, they "had" to drink heavily, both patriotic activities. This is an obvious medical oxymoron. Heavily drinking men are often impotent and unwilling to be sexually active in lieu of the more tangible habit of drinking. Under this mistaken ideology, men truly did become confused and passive-aggressive.

Russian men are stuck between the media's demand that they drink heavily to be macho and the low self-esteem and performance problems related to this behavior. Lost like this, they are despised by women whose expectations they cannot fulfill. Both genders are suspicious of each other, and more and more separated.

Men who are not alcoholics, despite the push from the state, are rare and are real heroes. Can you imagine the guts it takes to resist the everyday beer commercials telling you that you are a cool dude just because you are a man?! These men really shine. They are the last men of the Great Russia before the Revolution. They tap into a deeper Russianness and connect with Mendeleev, Dostoevsky, Tolstoy, Stravinsky, and Chagall. They drink silently from Russia's tradition of science, humanism, and art. Dr. Dmitry is certainly one of those exquisite men.

Gosha went to school number 239. So did Gregory Perelman: a true genius in mathematics, and a true eccentric. In 2002 Grisha (Gregory) solved the mathematical riddle that no mathematician had been able to solve for an entire century, the Poincare Conjecture. He was awarded all major mathematical prizes for his solution, but rejected them. He became a hero of many writers. Masha Gessen's brilliant book about Gregory Perelman is one.

What she wrote about the culture in the 239th helped me understand something about Gosha, too. It was something

I had felt and experienced for many years, but only now could I see the roots of his inability to engage in a dialogue with me. By definition of the Leningrad's Specialized Mathematics School Number 239 culture that formed these boys, made them feel superior for their mathematical rigor, a woman was an inferior creature. Perelman was surrounded by teachers who were more like coaches as they trained their charges for the competitive arena of mathematics and elite thought. His main mentor-coach was very happy that Grisha did not spend time on girls because this would distract him from mathematics and high-brow thinking, the only thing worth doing in life.

It was a culture inspired and instigated by Kolmogorov, a mathematician and scientist who was allowed to practice his science because it was useful for the Soviet Defense Systems. Mathematicians were needed to calculate the trajectories of rockets. Thus, mathematics was allowed to exist, untouched by ideology. That is how the division originated. Mathematics was perceived as useful; the rest of the world was not worth noticing.

All the Russian drinking mess was not allowed into this Castle of mathematics, logics and elitism. Perhaps this is why everything was so easy for these boys – they felt like they were above the rest of Russia, and that gave them a lot of power and invincibility. These boys lived in the land of possibilities, they exercised their brain with mathematics at school, and they were loved, cherished, adored at home. The privileged of the privileged, condescending to the rest of the world, and ready for action. Many of these math boys later became the Russian oligarchs, quickly figuring out the mathematics of post-Soviet economic success. But only those with guts, luck and perseverance. But not all. But all are still keeping the feeling of invincible condescension to the rest of the world. They already won, when they were these school boys. Don't dare to question and compete with the eternal victory.

But women survived anyway, men or no men, and carried through. They worked in the "damned 90's." They raised their families on their meager incomes, they studied, they adapted and got second degrees and new professions. They were the most active force in the society, but they were hated for that by the same society as too "manly."

**DEDICATION &
CERTIFICATION OF
THANKS TO:**

*Tara O. Frank,
L.OM.*

**ANNA THANKS YOU FOR
YOUR KIND SUPPORT!**

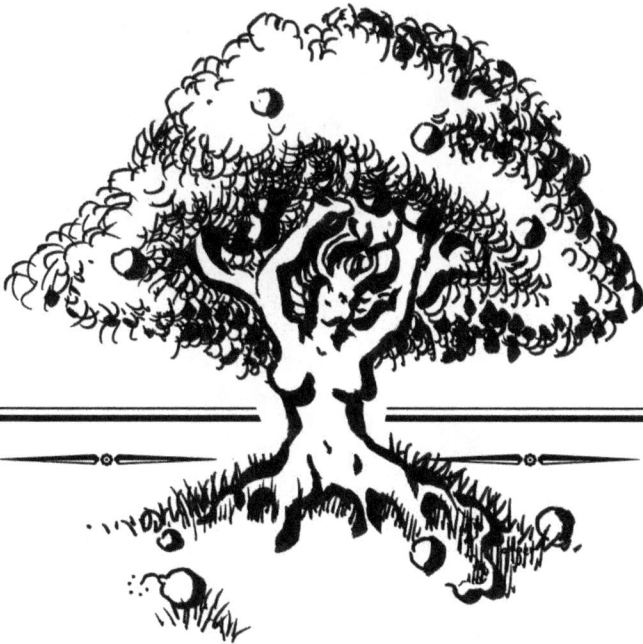

CHAPTER 33

Cell Count

I did one round of chemo with Dr. Chaikin, after which my white blood cell count plummeted. I was not allowed to have the next chemo treatment until it was back up again. By that time, I was feeling really good. I had no hair, I was very slender (which was great) and full of energy. Since I read in Lance Armstrong's memoirs about him riding every day, Gosha bought me a bicycle. Wearing a helmet on my bald head was a bit dramatic, so I put a knit cap on, under the helmet The whole neighborhood was very surprised to see a deathly ill cancer patient happily riding a bicycle!

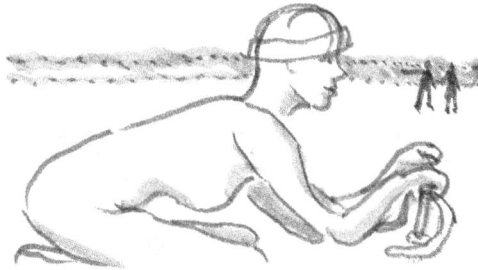

Happy as I was, I wanted to continue with chemo, thinking it very important to do without interruption. I don't know where I got this idea, but I adamantly stuck to it. When Terry, Dr. Chaikin's nurse, explained at length that my white blood cell count was still too low for my next treatment, I became very upset. I thought it was very important to continue chemo. Of course she sounded upbeat. "Don't worry Ms. Gutkina. Give it a week and your count will go back up by itself."

By then I had an aversion towards this upbeat tone. I knew she was not sure it was going to happen. I felt bad for Terry because I knew I was going to keep asking her questions and that she would not be able to answer because she was not a doctor. As weeks passed and the count was still low, I started to worry. A friend of mine, Annette, had undergone chemo the year before with Dr. Carrie Zizek. She was taking medicine to boost her immune cell count, stimulating immune cells to mature in the bone marrow. One shot cost seven thousand dollars.

"Can I get Neulasta?" I asked the nurse. "Neulasta and Neupogene? Whatever. To induce my immune cells like other people do?"

The nurse, Terry, was reluctant. I could not understand the roots of this tremendous reticence.

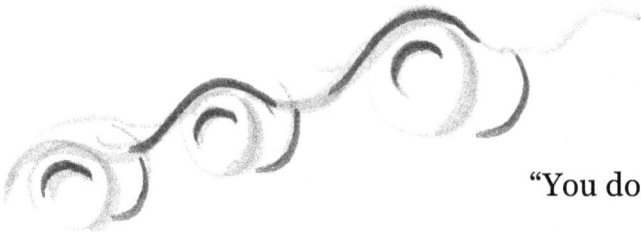

"You don't need it."

"But I was waiting for the immune cell count to go back to normal for my next chemo... How long now? Three weeks! And you promised one week!"

"No, Anna. I did not promise one week."

"Terry, I remember it very well. You said 'one week.'"

"Okay, I will ask the doctor."

"But I thought you have already asked the doctor."

"I did."

"And what did he say?"

"You don't really need Neulasta before the chemo because chemo is going to wipe out the immune cells, anyway. It is a long lasting drug."

"What do I need then?"

"You need Neupogene."

"Why?"

"Because it is more short-lived and you can take a shot of it every day."

"Then give me Neupogene?"

"I will ask the doctor and get back to you in a couple of days."

I would wait for another couple of days. Then, exhausted, I would brave a call.

"What did the doctor say?"

"That Neualasta would not really work for you, anyway."

"Why? It works for other people. Give me Neupogene."

"I will ask the doctor."

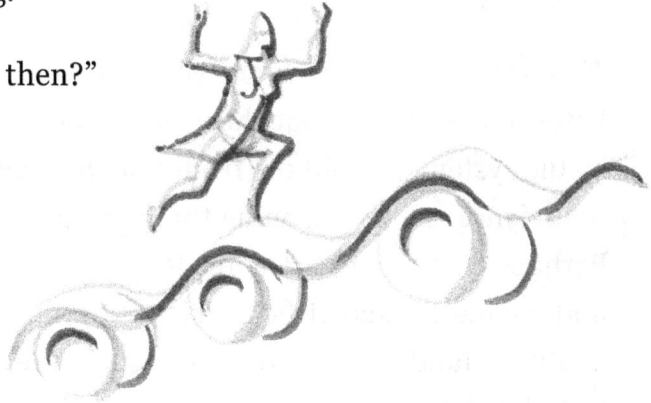

"No, Terry! Don't hang up! I have waited to continue my chemo for three weeks. This is the only way. What is the problem?"

"No problem."

"If you can't give me Neulasta, then give me Neupogene."

This was typical of my many conversations with poor Terry. Later, I understood that she was put there by the doctors, or by the system, to hold the front line. She could not explain the science or the reasoning that a doctor might have had. Perhaps doctors did not consider her smart enough to understand the scientific explanations and this made her unable to hold conversations with intelligent patients who would insist on intelligent treatment. Everyone in this field was so busy non-answering questions and non-concentrating on each particular case, that it left no time to think. On this conveyor belt, my pleas for attention had no chance of being heard.

I called Glenn. He had offered to accompany me to any appointment, if I wanted. This time, I took him up on his offer and we went to see Nurse Terry. As a teacher of Buddhism and equanimity, Glenn would be a perfect mediator. He had a calm ability to listen and relate to all humans involved in a conflict and this Neulasta/Neupogen situation looked like a ripening conflict to me. Glenn was unabashed. Unfortunately, it made no difference.

Finally, I had to write a letter to Dr. Chaikin. When I re-read it now, it looks hysterical and illogical, although I vividly remember spending a long time re-reading and rewriting it again and again before I impatiently hit the fatalistic "send" button.

Poor Dr. Chaikin must have been utterly confused by all the blood-dripping emotion I infused in the message, if he ever read it with full attention. He is such a patient and almost unnaturally calm doctor that all my justi-fied-by-my-dire-condition drama faded under his imper-vious calm. I had the sense he was smiling inside at all our interactions, eye-to-eye.

CHAPTER 34
In Vitro

While I was in Philadelphia, waiting for the next chemo appointment, going to meditation classes, remembering how to write, living fully, I got the news from Dr. Dmitry delivered in a way a Gogol's character would do it: "I have overly disappointing news..."

Dr. Dmitry wrote to me: "Anya, I have unpleasant news. We don't have enough cells. I started to grow them in vitro. They stopped growing after several divisions. Maybe they were affected by the chemo." The usual protocol included just cells from the tumor, this time it was already modified to get more cells by growing them in vitro. But there were still not enough cells. As Nabokov said about his alter ego prince... "What should we do?"

Obviously, it was time for the second batch of my cells. I called my genius cell biologist friend, David, who knew how to grow any cells from any source and they would not die but continue to divide. He was versed in growing stem cells. And stem cells are a reluctant bunch to just start dividing in your average Petri dish, stubborn little buds of the cells.

"Don't worry," he said. "If I could even grow these buds of a cells from a dead animal, I could certainly get some live cells from your pleural effusion liquid." And laughed. I loved that and felt that I was protected. There was the warm feeling of being in good hands again.

He already tried my cells in a secret medium in which even the least viable cells could grow. This was how we produced more cells for my vaccine. "Don't worry! We'll get them!" And later: "Your cells are growing well. I have them under control," David told me. "Do everything you need to. Don't worry about anything. Take care of yourself and your family. Love each other."

A true artist of cell growth he had a rare "oneness" with nature he lovingly watched and was thus capable of tricking into his own experiments. He was one of those mathematicians from the Castle of privileged mathematical thought himself, however belonging to the previous, less spoiled and less cherished generation than the generation of the perpetual boys. He was married to a talented cell biologist, a powerful researcher and a passionate wife and mother to their son. They were empowering each other, it seemed. And the fruits of their mutual non-contested relationships were many discoveries. Her enthusiasm and love for biology were so contagious, that he dropped his mathematical studies and turned his gaze to biology. He never read many papers, but he just thought about any particular process. And in his thinking, he just asked simple childish questions on the mechanics of a process, and then would search for answers, either in the literature, or in a test tube, until they could be answered one by one. Einstein did not have a lab. "My husband's lab is his head," his wife is known saying. Indeed, he ran the experiments in his mind also.

I felt myself being held in the warm and loving hands of a kind and knowledgeable power. It was one of the points in my journey were I could stop, catch a breath and relax.

These little breaks in life are so important and they show you the world loves you. I realized, once again, how fortunate I was that I was surrounded by people to whom my life mattered. The unforgettable faces of these people are assembled into a virtual portrait gallery in my head now. I want to say thank you to those who of you who gave me this wonderful chance to think and to be.

THANK YOU!

CHAPTER 35
Contribution

A friend's wife, Nonna, was about to go to Russia for her birthday. Gosha asked her to take my cells for the Russian vaccine with her. She said "yes" at first, then she said "no." Gosha talked to her, and delivered a tearful explanation of her unfortunate refusal: Nonna's airplane had too short of a connection in Paris. We did not understand how the length of a layover affected her ability to carry the flasks. Gosha was very upset, as he always was when people declined to help. He ended relationships over this sort of refusal. He could not even remotely understand why people might not be able to help. But I learned, by then, not to dwell on disappointments but to move on quickly. I would have forgotten about Nonna if Gosha hadn't kept bringing it up, nodding his head in disbelief. "No," he would say,"I don't get it. The stopover is too short... And then what?!" But a couple of days later he came home shining and happy:

"She was sitting at the synagogue and she decided that she needs to do a mitzvah!"

"What? Who?" I asked

"She is taking it!" He continued to shine. "Nonna is taking it! It is a mitzvah!"

Then the wheels started to turn. Priding himself as a logistics genius, Gosha was back in the game. It was time for him to go into action and organize yet another shipment to

Russia. The growth factors and the medium were ordered, mixed and driven to Nonna. Much to Gosha's delight, all his plans went smoothly and, upon collecting the flasks from Nonna at the airport, my father quickly delivered the medium to the lab. Gosha became another one of my saviors, a very important one and as indispensable as the rest of them. The chain of saviors that could not be broken. He became a link in this chain, a true manager of operations. And a very efficient one. Because the operation was a success!

Gosha organized the meeting of Nonna and my Dad in Saint Petersburg. I was really spared from all these managerial decisions. Gosha made all the calls, connected all the flights, "Your father is so cute, so... noble. Say 'Hi' to him!" Nonna and her husband would always mention my father, whenever we would talk. My father knows how to wear his suits in style, always did. It is so unusual for a Russian man of his age, that my friends were always impressed. In fact, he liked style so much, that style found him. He became a machinist at first, then somebody like a CEO of a factory in Saint Petersburg that made men's suits and coats. He grew the factory from an old Soviet era enterprise that made low quality suits into a modern one that made suits famous for their good cut and quality. People's favorite men's suits were made in Saint Petersburg, at his factory. He was smart, loved by workers, and quickly rose to an executive position after the beginning of perestroika. And to think that he had never pursued this type of work! My father had been a radio engineer in his first profession, but in order to feed his children (me and my brother), he had to take this new job. He had been fired from radio enginnering, and gazing at the lofty radio stars, for something like being too Jewish. I remember how I was crushed by his loss of his lofty status as a star-gazer. It was my identity, and then it was gone overnight! And what was worst, he did not want to come anywhere near the star gazing ever again. I begged and pleaded but to no avail. He was stern in being unemployed for a long time, and then becoming what I called "just" a machinist. "Why can't you be a star-gazer again?" I would demand at our kitchen table discussion that had seen happier dialogues between a status father and adoring daughter. More like lectures about everything, including the beauty of the German language.

"I just can't," I remember him saying to my angry astonishment.

"BUT WHY?!"

"I just can't" he would say over and over again.

"But you are so smart! Come on!"

"I told you. I just can't."

I did not yet know that he had this success story ahead of him that would happen later. But from back then it was exactly like it is now between me and my children when they ask the same question:

"Mom, why don't you take a corporate job!"

And the answer would be the same. It is wonderful how our past keeps repeating itself in our future families.

No escape, only hopes that this time around it will be a softer landing, and a more solid success, and a little bit more celebration, and little bit more love. Not radically, but a notch better.

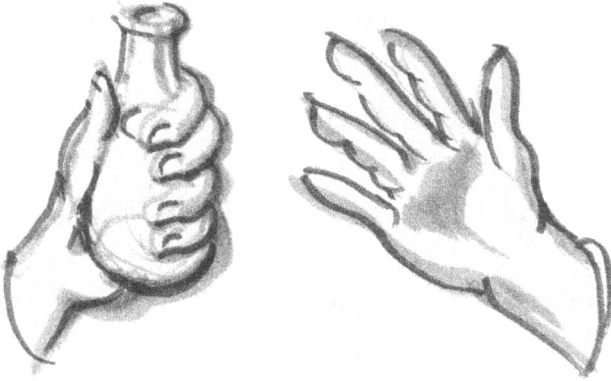

When it was time for my son to graduate from middle school, and he needed a suit for the graduation ceremony, the last suit he had was too small. I bought it when he was a tiny little boy of ten, and it didn't fit the twelve year old slim giant he had become. It was, of course, the evening before the event when Simon let us know about it. We had no choice but to dig into Gosha's wardrobe. There it was: the suit Gosha wore for his high school graduation and that he brought with him all the way to America. It had hung untouched in that closet for twenty years. This suit was made at my dad's factory during the time when he was still just a mechanic there. Now, his grandson was wearing it. Of course, the suit did not quite fit. It was an old world creation, made according to old standards and with materials that are now used only in a very expensive personalized tailoring: a handshake from my father's past.

When Nonna brought my materials for the vaccine and
my father met her at the airport, polite and stylish in his
factory's suit and the coat, ready to deliver it to Dr. Dmitry,
he was just a humble man trying to save his daughter. Now,
I did not have to worry about a shortage of antigen for my
vaccine, and just had to wait for my next visit to Russia.
Now, my vaccine would be completed with more than
the desired amount of cells. Thanks to all my friends who
contributed to the project—from the fluid extraction and
the stimulation of cell growth, to the flask preparation, the
transportation logistics and the actual travel—the cell base
for my antigen was now stronger than had we been able to
use the tumor itself.

CHAPTER 36

Side Effects

I was told I would need at least eight cycles of chemo. I was determined to do them all. I had completed one infusion of carboplatin and taxol, intravenously. Then, I had transferred to the University of Pennsylvania and completed a cycle of bi-monthly infusion: a complex protocol including one abdominal "chemo wash" with cisplatin with simultaneous intravenous infusion of taxol. That was followed, three weeks later, by a simpler session of intravenous infusion of cisplatin. The abdominal part of the treatment is called IP, for intra-peritoneal, and was only made available to me by Dr. Chaikin at the University of Pennsylvania.

No other doctor from any other hospital even mentioned that option to me. Not Fox Chase, Jefferson, Sloan Kettering, let alone the local Hope Memorial. I am surprised that, after its official recommendation by the NIH to oncologists and gynecologists in 2006, the intra-peritoneal protocol was only offered to me by one doctor.

From the web site of Harvard medical school (http://www. health.harvard.edu/newsweek/Abdominal_chemotherapy_improves_ovarian_cancer_survival.htm):

> *Based on the results of eight trials in the past*
> *two decades (sic!) comparing intravenous*
> *(by vein) chemotherapy with a combination*
> *of intravenous and IP therapies, the National*
> *Cancer Institute issued an alert in January 2006*

encouraging clinicians to use IP therapy after surgery for ovarian cancer.

I don't wonder why it took so long. I know the answer.

The announcement coincided with the publication of a study in the Jan. 5, 2006, New England Journal of Medicine, *reporting that women with newly diagnosed ovarian cancer who received chemotherapy drugs directly into the abdomen (see graphic) lived 16 months longer than women who got standard intravenous chemotherapy — the longest increase in survival time reported in any randomized trial for ovarian cancer.*

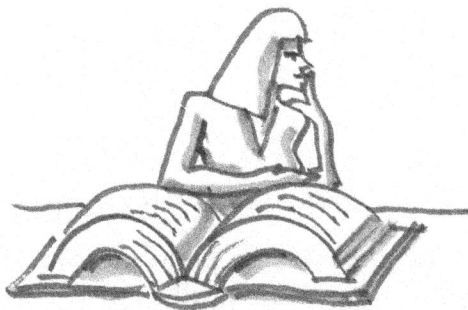

It benefits an average doctor not to risk excellence. Being slow to adopt new treatments does not present any risk to their careers.

Although the women who received part of their chemotherapy by abdomen survived longer, many found the treatment extremely difficult. IP therapy improves outcomes in part because higher doses of the drugs can be used. But side effects include severe fatigue, pain, infections, and gastrointestinal and neurological problems.

I did not experience much of anything like that at all. I expected much worse and was surprised when none of my worst fears came true. Especially in the beginning, I felt hardly any discomfort. Even the absence of hair turned out to be an opportunity to experiment with wigs.

I also feel that meditation and all my alternative medical experimentation made a difference. I am surprised, reading other people's accounts of their side effects. It was only after being disease-free for a year that I went though a time of feeling extremely toxic and began to have problems with my blood pressure, and just felt that I was deteriorating. But, I'll get to that later.

> *Catheter-related complications were also*
> *a problem.*

Once, only once, was there some leaking from the port site, or rather it was leaking from my abdomen through the port after the chemotherapy solution was administered. It was almost funny because I had to go to Russia in two days, and the only fear I had was that I would miss my trip. I asked my nurses, who were more worried than I was:

"Will I be able to fly in two days?"

They weren't sure and they told me they would ask the doctor.

"Yes," they came back, "if we can stop this leak."

"Is it a big deal? Will you?"

"We'll stop it. No problem."

And they did.

"Just call us if it leaks again."

I was done. Hence this was the only scary episode, or near scary.

Because of the story that I am about to tell, I was able to tolerate chemotherapy treatments very well. The story goes like this: Once, there was a Russian-Jewish woman who had married a Chinese man in the 1950's or early 1960's and they had a son. The Chinese-Soviet relationship deteriorated, and the husband had to go to China leaving his son and wife behind. In the 1990's, the family immigrated to the US. The woman got cancer and had troubles tolerating chemo.

After learning the news, her former husband, who was now married to a Chinese woman and living in China, insisted that she follow the traditional Chinese recommendation of herbal teas. The prescribed mixture of herbs was shipped to her for the duration of her chemotherapy, which she survived. Later, the woman had a recurrence and had to undergo chemo again. This time the herbs were not available, for some reason. Unfortunately, she had to stop chemotherapy altogether because of side effects. She later died.

This woman's son is somehow related to Gosha's friend Kolya, and through his Chinese family there came a connection to a famous Chinese medicine doctor in New York. We rushed to him right before chemo and bought a lot of herbs, enough to for me to make teas for a couple of months. He was a calm man who looked at my tongue, at my palms, felt the pulse, looked me into the eyes and said, through the woman interpreter: "You are fine. Just relax. Don't drink. Eat well. Go for walks. Relax." It was like a mantra to me that I have repeated in my head for a long time since then.

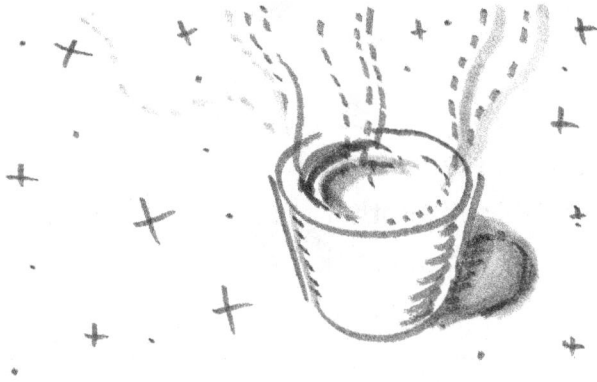

He gathered five or more types of different seeds, fruits and herbs from the little drawers in his store. We immediately went to a Chinese restaurant he recommended and ate a soup with a huge mushroom in it. At first, Gosha diligently cooked the herbs. Herbs were given to me in a small lunch paper bags, a mix of serpentine fruits, dried grasses, slices of wood. A special ceramic teakettle was bought at a nearby store in Chinatown in New York City. The herbs were soaked in a couple liters of water, then boiled for an hour until only a cup of liquid remained. The tea was now dark and smelly. Then, more fresh water was added, the herbs were boiled again for another hour. Then, they were strained again, and two products combined.

I drank one cup at night and heated up the second one in the morning. The smell was quite horrible, by my children's account, and "earthy" by Glenn's. My mother, who lived with us in the US for whole time I was doing chemo, took over the duty of cooking the Chinese tea, filling the air with a secret earthy smell ancient as the world. Maybe because of these herbs, I too tolerated chemo quite well. Actually, when I stopped drinking these teas, after my mother left for Russia, I did start to feel the side effects of chemo. I should have continued to drink them.

Going to New York City was a bit too hard, and soon I found another herbalist in Philly. My friend and cancer guru Annette shared another person from her "cancer network" – it was Cara Frank. Cara's office in Center City was a stark difference to the Chinese Doctor's in China town. I am a person who can be sold on design, and I was sold immediately. I was sold when I saw a witty combination of the same medicinal chests from the Metropolitan Museum, posters from the Maoist China, and a Center City Philadelphia modest modern look. I came to the office with Glenn and we waited in Cara's witty waiting room for her consultation, acupuncture and mercy.

I kept thinking those design thoughts when Cara buzzed into the waiting room – she was busy with two other conversations, handing the jar with some pills to another patient, checking something in her journal, talking to her receptionist, and shouting somewhere into the basement the details about the next patient's herbs, and cheerfully took me into the gust of her office.

More design, I thought with almost a sigh of relief – everything was so cool. Cara sat me down near the desk and started taking notes.

"So," Cara said, "I am taking notes. Let's start from the beginning."

And I told her everything from the beginning, feeling as always apologetic for the overburdening length of my story and the details of the gory discoveries. Doctors telling me I was doomed. I was ready for the familiar "Oh-sorry –to hear in what deep shit you are."

"Well," Cara said instead , "There was a woman here who everybody said was doomed. Like a year they gave her. We took her in. We found her a good doctor."

I felt I was not a burden but a curious case for improvement.

"And?"

"Well, she had five nice years. Nice years."

"Yeah," I agreed, "that's a lot." And I thought about how much it was – five years.

Cara's message was that it was not the end – but an opportunity to improve my situation.

She too observed my tongue, eyes, and pulse.

"You are dry," she announced. "Too much wind. We'll work on your kidneys."

She took me to one of the procedure rooms, I undressed and she inserted the needles.

"We'll work on improving your immune system, your mood and obviously your kidney. Chemo dries you out. Just relax."

I laid there with the needles all over my body, fighting with the desire to fall asleep, I felt so sleepy, and I think I dozed off. It was against my "principles" of a strong person, but I succumbed.

I would see Cara a lot after that. I became a regular. Her non-drama approach was healing in itself.

I would see her a lot in between my trips to Russia. I would lay there under the sheets with needles sticking out of my body, succumbing to the dream of wellness and calm. Unashamed of being cared for. Unashamed of being weak and sick.

"And when you are done – step out and I will give you some herbs for moisture."

On my way out I would get the lunch bags with some herbs—similar to the Chinese doctor from New York – and some pills—melatonin, probiotics for the digestive tract, and other herbs, lots of herbs. I would leave rested, relieved of my worries and loaded with herbs.

Making the herb tea—oh my God how it smelled!—was a chore for my Mom, Gosha, and me. It was the true year of herbs. I still have a couple of lunch bags that I did not use, and I still have the dark brown ceramic teakettle in my kitchen.

But I think this battle against the "Chinese wind" helped me a lot to sustain my health during what appears to be a very strong chemo regiment.

As Dr. Chaikin has said, I was strong and I could sustain

a lot of chemo. Namely the twice a month combination
of intra-peritoneal infusions and intravenous injections.
Strong stuff. Was I strong? I don't know. But I was relaxed
and drinking Chinese herbs. And that helped.

> *Nearly 6 in 10 of the women in the IP group
> switched partway through the trial to standard
> intravenous chemotherapy. Yet those women
> survived longer than the intravenous-only
> group. This suggests that even some IP therapy
> is better than none at all — and that greater
> benefits may be likely if it can be made more
> tolerable. In the meantime, the National Cancer
> Institute is advising physicians to discuss IP
> therapy with newly diagnosed women who
> are candidates for the treatment and to refer
> patients to centers that offer it if their own
> institutions do not.*

I was not looking for this treatment. I met Dr. Chaikin
because I was looking for immunotherapy. This happens so
often, in life: we are looking for one thing, but find another.
I appointed Dr. Chaikin "my doctor" and thought he would
have time and capacity to do all the things I wanted from
him, but this was not possible. It is a popular illusion
that we can get everything from one person. My lesson to
myself, yet again, was not to overwhelm the good people I
meet on my journeys with every responsibility and expect
them to solve to all my problems.

CHAPTER 37
The Russian Egg

Glenn encouraged me to continue writing. I had been scribbling all my life and, after moving to America, had been writing what I thought would be a long novel about a young Russian woman in America. It would be based on my own life and on all the funny stories I'd gathered from my female friends. But, during that winter of pre-diagnosis devastation and failed expectations—What a big deal! I should have just gotten new ones!—I stopped writing. When I was admitted to the hospital with a stroke, I made a promise to myself that, if I survived, I would write, only write.

Glenn decided I should start writing, immediately. I was a little peevish, but Glenn pushed on, asking me for more and more material. We discussed how much of the original voice we should leave. I came to the US when I was 28. Having an accent, for me, was always part stigma and part intellectual trademark. It was also a bit of a relief to write in English. In Russian, I would agonize over each word, sometimes for hours, sometimes fruitlessly. I was ambitious and would struggle towards uncompromisingly "non-cliché" phrasing. Sometimes the result would be sharp and weird and fresh, but the effort was enormous. In English, I don't have the luxury of fluency, so I simply focus on being clear. One day, when I have more time for writing, I will find the magic Russian-English dictionary that Vladimir Nabokov used to come up with the flavor of his language.

Writing drafts for Glenn was good for me. It was a fun

project that gave me a lot of energy and the feeling that it could be done. My friends Curt Dilger and Mark Khaisman, both architect-artists, even illustrated it for me! The book was called *The Russian Egg*. The cover was red and, on the front page, it had an egg with wings that did not look like chicken egg but looked rather like a male testicle. The red background symbolized the Soviet era, the vignette in the middle symbolized the Russia of the 19th century, and the testicles were a reference to the feministic battles that constituted the book's content. It felt extraordinary to see myself through the the eyes of American men: as a ballsy Russian Bond girl with no fear. I was very proud.

Accomplishing this small project, a little twenty five page kitten of a book, gave me so much creative energy and drive to continue that I did another writing project. This time, I collected all the stories that I ever wrote in Russian. My distant cousin Katia Asmus organized the publication of a book that featured my stories. In Russia, people were interested in America and what it feels like to be there. So, I wrote about my first car, a 1970's Oldsmobile. I wrote about car culture, about psychotherapy culture, and about everything American. When the book was published in Russia, I got my fifteen minutes of fame and even a poet admirer who followed me everywhere. He drank heavily and recited the poetry of Mandelshtam and Blok. He even proposed to marry me but, of course, it was a joke. He was very patriotic and bohemian at the same time, and he drank vodka at his friend's studios, formerly bohemian but now lost drunks, former members of the once powerful Union of the Soviet Artists. It was a time machine back to the Soviet era, a secret passage to the times when salaried poets were given the ticket to insanity. I was presented, semi-romantically, as an American girl. I was wearing my blond wig and nobody had any idea about my cancer or about my baldness, or about the Russian vaccine. I came across as a successful writer living in America, calm, happy, sleek, undoubtedly rich, and perhaps worth consideration. This was an even bigger boost to my self-esteem.

Since I was going to Russia every month for my vaccine, I spent a lot of time in Saint Petersburg. Katia organized several public readings in the exceptionally cold winter of 2009. One time, when I landed—I think it was January of 2009, or perhaps February—I went to Saint Petersburg to celebrate my birthday. Saint Petersburg struck me, on that visit, in perhaps the way it strikes foreigners: as pure magic. It was incredibly cold. Snow covered the sidewalks, the roads, the canals, the roofs, the parks, the trees, the window sills, the columns, the porticos, the statues, the steps of the stairwells, the broad Neva river, the bridges, the street lamp poles. I took a taxi from the tiny airport across the city to Vasilevsky Ostrov. The taxi drivers smoking outside would hop to keep their blood flowing. It was the type of cold that causes birds to fall from the sky like bricks. I got into the warmth of a car and watched the frozen city unravel before my eyes, as if for the first time.

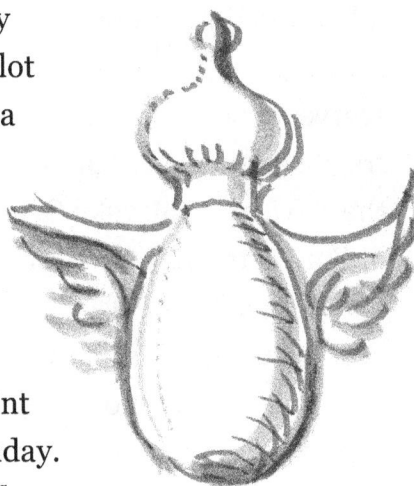

After a fifteen minute drive through a 1960's Moskovsky Highway, we entered the old city. Sadovya Square, destroyed once and lately remodeled but still surrounded by a few old buildings, a backdrop of Dostoevsky's and Gogol's novels, was all frozen in a quiet winter smog. Smoke rose slowly from the roofs. Without wind, the smoke waited silently in the air, as if encased in the opalescent glass bubble that was the city of Saint Petersburg.

I would not have been surprised if people had chosen to hibernate through this cold, but they were walking and working and breathing out little clouds of warm air through scarves covering their noses and mouths. The city was as fragile as an icicle, but alive and functioning. We crossed the Neva to Vasilevsky Ostrov. Here was the Academy of Fine Arts whose first president Ekaterina Dashkova had been a friend of Voltaire and Franklin. Her formerly best friend, Ekaterina the Great, sent her into exile. Two Egyptian Sphinxes overlooked the river, dreamy under caps of snow. A man swept the sidewalks. Then the doors of a church opened and happily chattering bundles spilled out in twos and threes. At this moment, I realized why foreigners were so fascinated with Russia. They must have seen it at one of these moments when human resilience overcame the impossible natural conditions and people rose above it to go about their usual business. I can imagine some Italians crying out: "How? What? In this cold? They are actually living?!!!" The insides of houses are always kept very warm. You just have to rush to your destination and relax inside, opening up to the extreme warmth and comfort.

I spent my days in Saint Petersburg going to poetic hangouts and art studios, to concerts and nice restaurants, making my way through the snow, avoiding icicles threatening to fall on my poor wigged head, balancing on the sidewalks between piles of snow, dodging the Tajik workers who slaved nobly to make the city livable through the tough winter. I went to a party at a flat where it is believed Nastasia Fillipovna from Dostoevsky's *Idiot* was killed by her jealous lover. I walked near the *Crime and Punishment* murder scene. I went to Mariinski Theater and the Mariinsky Concert Hall. Its director, Gergiev, inspired the cultural life of Saint Petersburg with his theater. I saw beautiful performances, some staged by the best Western choreographers and opera directors.

For the first time in my life, I was sold on Russia. I had lived in this same city all my life in this same cold and hated it: the cold, the cold, the cold. But now I was sold, perhaps like the Italian architect who built Saint Petersburg in the 18th century, or like the French dancer who started the Russian Ballet. I was so sold that I did not want to leave this country. I wanted to observe the people. I wanted to get some of their resilience and their hard armor. They seemed like superior beings because they could survive in cold and snow.

CHAPTER 38
Taxol

I was so scared by one of the doctors at UPenn, Dr. Bajusz, that I agreed to participate in one very strange clinical trial that at first seemed kind of stupid to me. But wait... He was substituting for Dr. Chaikin that day.

— I —

"Congratulations patient Gutkina! You are doing really well," he told me when I reported in. It was after I finished my eight cycles of bimonthly chemos, around month 10 since my diagnosis. They always said that to me: "Congratulations!" It was probably supposed to be uplifting, but it sounded like they were surprised I was still alive.

"Thanks," I said, shy as a bride.

"Your disease is horrible, you know that, right?" said Dr. Bajusz.

"Aahm..."

"Yes, your disease is horrible."

"Okay. What are you suggesting?" I asked.

"Well, let's see. There is a clinical trial that you need to participate in. Your disease is horrible."

His English was rather simplistic, perhaps because he

thought I was only able to comprehend very rudimentary phrases. Indeed he was not that far from the truth because my stroke and followed by 8-9months of chemo made me what they call "chemo-brained." It took me a while to realize that. I was told he was from Hungary. I lived in Hungary as part of the Young Scientists UNESCO program, and I love this country. I scrambled my language memories together and greeted him in Hungarian:

"Yonapotkivanook."

"What?"

"Yonapotkivanok."

He was so surprised, that he did not get it the first time.

"It is Hungarian," I said. "I lived in Szeged for a year."

"Oh great! What were you doing there?"

We had a nice conversation. He told me was going to the Soviet Union for some extreme travel in the mountains of Uzbekistan or Tajikistan, and that he loved it. I liked this about Dr. Bajusz, and immediately trusted him. I forgave him his clumsy English and his simplistic approach to English. I thought, wouldn't it be nice to have him as a potential partner in my future immunotherapy company... I find courage to be a very rare condition and I immediately like it when I see it. So I liked him. American thought requires a different kind of courage, and this was something I was curious to find out. He convinced me bravely to bravely go for the additional chemotherapy. I regretted it at first. But now I am not sure it was not a right thing. But back then it was a difficult decision. I just started growing my hair back, and would now be facing the prospect of losing it again due to chemo.

"Okay," I said. "What is it?"

"I am glad," he said. "Let's arrange your appointment with Dr. Howe, who is in charge of this trial."

I decided to do the clinical trial that was another chemotherapy drug for 12 months, under the mantra, "Your disease is horrible" and "aren't you brave."

✦ II ✦

Dr. Howe was very upfront.

"Doing this trial, you will get the benefit of disease free progression."

"What is that?"

"This is the period when you will have no disease."

"Okay. And, how about... mmm... how long will I live?"

"Life expectancy is the same."

I was struck by these two facts. They made no sense to me.

"So, why would I want to do it?"

"You will get the benefit of disease free progression."

"But life expectancy is not longer?"

"True. But you will get the benefit of the disease free progression."

He continued: "You will be getting the new drug for twelve months."

"Okay. Will I lose my hair?"

"No. That is, if you get into the branch that gets it."

"What do you mean?"

He explained something I had sort of already known that, in the blind randomized trials, one branch of patients receives the drug and the other two receive standard therapy: in this case, taxol.

"Then I will lose my hair if I am not in this branch."

"Yes."

"What are the chances that I end up in the taxol branch?"

"We have no control over it. That's up to the designers of the trial. But there is a chance that we can get the drug, here."

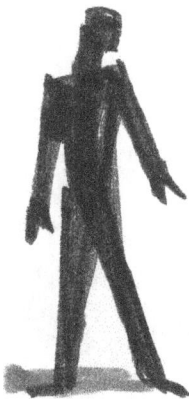

He sent me over to Nurse Kathy who was responsible for conducting clinical trials and all the paper work that was associated with the process. I signed up and was waiting for the result of the lottery which would tell me in which branch I would be. The lottery was played somewhere in the guts of the NIH. After a while, I got the result: I was not in the new drug branch, but I could take a low dose of taxol for twelve months.

Needless to say, I was devastated. My hair was growing and I did not want to wear a wig for another twelve months. I had had enough fun with wigs, by then. In my usual combative style, I wrote a letter to Dr. Chaikin demanding to put me in the "real" branch. I don't think he even replied.

At that time I stumbled upon several successful accounts of women who were still around and posting on the ovarian cancer message board. I forced myself to read some of them. A post would go like this: "I want to encourage all those women... I did chemotherapy such and such... And I am still here." I noticed a strong common motif among survivors: they all spent longer than the usual five to eight months in chemotherapy. I calculated that success stories reported a full year of chemotherapy. This was a compelling reason for me to undergo additional chemotherapy. Finally, I gave up and said, "Yes."

My latest basic eight month chemo started October 2nd. I started the low dose of taxol in December. It was supplemented with avastin. That made some sense. Avastin had been part of a treatment that had been dangled before me as a possible clinical trial but, due to how recently I had had a stroke, it was not recommended at that time.

I pulled my wigs out of the closet and went bald again.

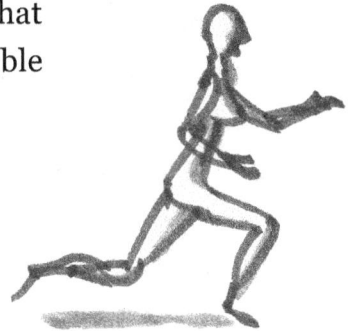

However, by the third chemo session, I felt so incredibly bad that I decided to quit after the forth one. As always, after each chemotherapy session, I would go to Russia for my Russian vaccine. After the last session in April 2010, I had spent a solid year in chemotherapy. I did not feel well. I felt something I have never felt before: pulsation in my neck, not just noticeable but quite heavy. I couldn't fall asleep. I felt light and my heart was pounding. Walking down the street in Saint Petersburg with my father, we discussed the possibility that my heart rate might be high. We walked into a pharmacy and bought a device for measuring blood pressure and heart rate. I tried in the store. My heart rate was well above normal. My blood pressure upper level was at the 140 mark. I asked my father to look away. He did. He only asked: "Is it high?"

"Kind of," I said.

I bought the device and, when we got home, I checked my heart rate and blood pressure yet again. They were very high. I noticed that, when I panicked, the symptoms worsened. If I meditated, my heart rate and blood pressure would go down. It was amazing. I immediately contacted Dr. Chaikin and he recommended a type of blood pressure medication that was available at Saint Petersburg pharmacies. I took it for several months. When I returned to the US for my appointment with Dr. Chaikin, we decided to stop chemo: "High blood pressure and no impact on life expectancy. Yeah. Let's discontinue treatment."

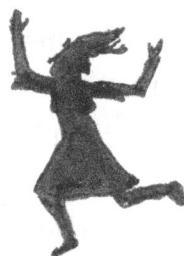

I continued to go to Russia for my dendritic vaccine every couple months, even though Dr. Dmitry wondered if I needed to continue. I insisted because I was scared. Also, my marriage was falling apart at home. So, I traveled.

CHAPTER 39
My Venice

When I got sick and thought I was about to die, I made a bucket list of things I would do if I survived. I remembered how I loved to travel. At first to Russia for the vaccine, then making a stopover in Paris a couple of times, Munich, and eventually flying myself to India and Italy. The world started to open up. I started to see the many ways people live and used to live. It was a different life.

❧ I ❧

I love Italy and have been there three times. I love it more and more every time I am there. The first time I went to Venice was with Sasha and five year old Simon. Three year old Naomi was left home, did not like it, and stopped eating. We actually had to cut the vacation short! Since then, the fact that Simon enjoyed Venice while Naomi was left home was a major sore point. Naomi complained to be taken to Italy, for years.

So, the first thing on my bucket list was to take Naomi to Italy. The summer after the chemo, we went. Naomi is a budding singer, so we went to Verona to see the opera at Arena de Verona. We froze there in the crisp August nights that fell so suddenly in the midst of simmering summer days. Naomi was very impressed, and remembered several arias. She is a natural. We visited Venice, drove to Rome, and then back to Milan.

 In Venice, we met many locals who were friendly in a typical Venetian way that is both miraculous and mundane at the same time. Walking down a narrow street, the kind where Casanova disappeared in the night from the Doge's police, we encountered a puff of expensive perfume and rushed to follow a group of finely dressed locals who were in quite a hurry. We followed them in the swirl of their luxurious smell, flying forward somewhere. We turned corners, keeping up, panting, even though Naomi was starting to grumble. "Mom, what are you doing?" I would just say, "Let's keep up!" She would sigh and throttle along. The group we had been following went into the open doors of a baroque theater, chirping like birds. We raced inside, trying to see. The ticket controller smiled at us, as if we too were legitimate: "Are you coming in?" We walked in.

It was a Russian-Italian cultural event, with a reception before the show. Tuvan dancers in ancient ornaments, with furs and fish skins, mingled with the audience. The Italian men wore suits, the Russian women smelled of luxurious perfumes. I was approached by a waiter with prosecco and

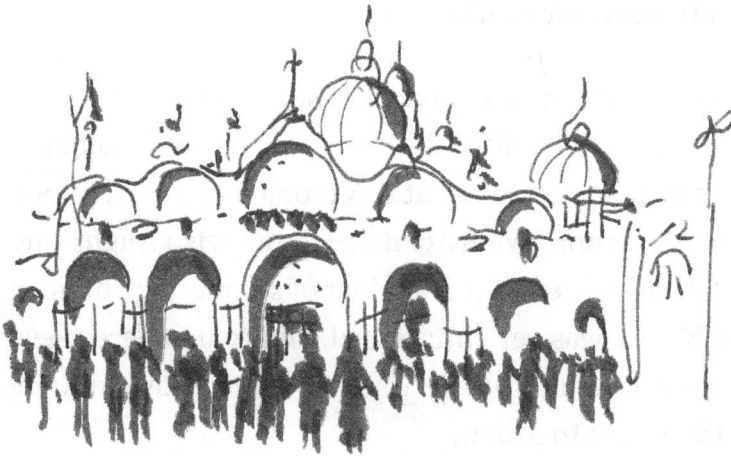

we started to make rounds around the room and that is
how we met Sveta, and two real, natural, organic Venetians:
Sveta's husband, Franko, and the artist Gianmaria.
Sveta, who happened to be a Professor of Russian at
the University of Venice, overheard our Russian and
approached us. We exchanged 'what-brought-you-here's',
translated into Italian by Sveta.

The very tall Franko laughed from his immense heights. He
did not speak Russian, nor did he speak any other language
than Italian. When Franko speaks, his meaning is so
obvious that I thought I knew Italian already. He looked
me in the eye and pronounced every word clearly and
profoundly, as if the word was living its own life. He would
nudge each one so patiently, as a parent would encourage a
shy child onto a stage to sing. His words did sing. Another
very tall Venetian dressed all in white with the Jean-Paul
Sartre-ian glasses and Leo Tolstoy's beard was introduced
to us as Gianmaria, an artist. He also spoke no other lan-
guages but Italian, but with Sveta's translating and Franko's
articulation, everybody was happy with the depth of
the conversation.

We were immediately invited to take a walk in Venice, to
stop for a drink, to visit Gianmaria's studio, and to dine at
Sveta's and Franko's. The next day we went for a walk in
Venice with Sveta and Franko. Having spent several days in
Venice, already, we thought we traversed every street. We'd
been scuttling about with tourist crowds, and were overwhelmed by the amount of beauty, culture, and artifacts of
humanity at its best. But now our beloved locals took us to
the quiet districts we'd never seen.

It was a hot summer day and wonderfully silent. A stranger like me could appreciate the empty canals and the beautiful facades of the palazzos while passing one palazzo after another. We stopped at the request of our guides, looked around and breathed it all in. The palazzos revealed little more than a hurried stranger would notice: the inner courtyards, the *gardini*, the secret lush flowers, trees, statues and gazebos, grapevines, Byzantine columns, Greek porticos, Persian statues and the ghosts of the Venetian Republic.

Franko knocked on a little door in the wall near the quiet canal. There was a long clicking and clacking of the old metal parts of a lock, then a young man opened and invited us in. It was a big yard with a hangar. Franko chatted with his friend. Sveta occasionally translated when she was not caught up in the conversation herself.

"How is business?"

"The Chinese are taking over."

"The Chinese are making Venetian gondolas?"

"Apparently."

"Will the young one take over your business?"

"I hope. My son is not interested though. This is just my apprentice. He might."

We went to the hangar and were allowed to touch a centuries old frame that is used for building a gondola.

"A Gondola must be a little curved, not straight as it seems to be, this is for stability. Hence the curve in the frame. My great-great-grandfather built this frame."

Everything had deep roots in this world. Casanova would have made his escape in one of the gondolas made in this ship yard.

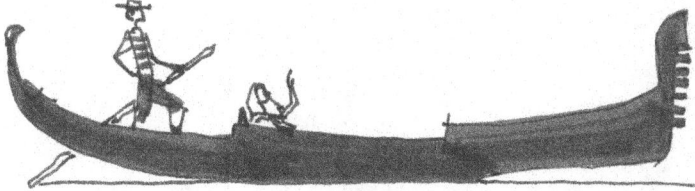

> II <

The next day, we visited the art studio of Gianmaria Potenza. We passed through a series of inner yards, little rooms, some modern, some very old. Dusty tools of some trade hung on the walls lined with ceramic tiles. Gianmaria had inherited this house from his father and grandfather, both craftsmen of Venice. The central garden was decorated with several metal sculptures by Gianmaria, himself. Some were primitive obelisks with geometric spikes. Others formed animals: a hippopotamus, a horse, an iron zoo. We sat down for prosecco, cookies and a chat in a modern study room.

"And what does the young lady do?"

"The young lady is a singer."

"Oh, nice to meet another artist. Let me give you my

books," and Gianmaria did a quick sketchy drawing as a way of signing this book for Naomi. She gracefully returned the favor by drawing something in return. Venice was full of magic.

"Come next year," said Gianmaria. "But you must learn to speak Italian."

"Sure," I said. "No problem. I promise."

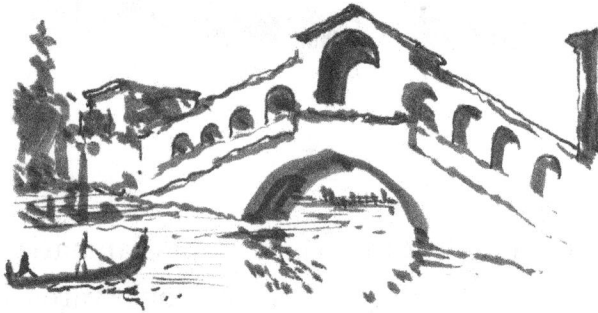

The next year came quickly. My next Italian trip was booked and fast approaching. I gave myself six weeks to master Italian after I booked the tickets. I wrote a letter to Gianmaria informing him that my friend Olga, an artist from Saint-Petersburg, and I were going to be in Venice on such and such a date. He wrote me back, and we decided to meet. I was using Google translate, thinking that I had enough time to learn some Italian.

I took Olga to see the Ducal palace and was crossing Piazza San Marco when I bumped into Gianmaria. I opened my mouth to say something and could not. I stood there with my mouth open trying to talk. He was waiting. We parted. I read in his eyes: "I told you to master Italian first, girl!" This is my resolution now: to learn Italian. There is something in it for me, I can feel it. But, somehow, I always forget!

This time, again, we met with Sveta and Franko, and went bar hopping along the Strada Nova where they live. We had dinner in their apartment, in a palazzo divided into apartments for the separate members of their growing family. We had a walk in the Jewish Ghetto. This was a tiny neighborhood, thick with buildings. It reminded me of my childhood neighborhood in Saint Peterburg were the same overcrowding resulted in the same solution. I was very surprised to see how similar the infamous "city courtyards" were: a small square area squished in between the sur-rounding four to five storied buildings. I could almost hear the loud voices yelling at the kids to stop their games and come in for lunch.

❧ III ❧

Cancer is called "the plague of the modern era." Indeed it has these elements of collective horror and tremendous loss. During the plague of 1630 in Venice, thirty percent of Venetians died. According to Wikipedia, forty six thousand people died within that year: one third of the Venice popu-lation, which had been a mere hundred and fifty thousand to start.

How many people die from cancer in the US, each year? Out of three hundred million people five hundred thousand die from cancer. It is less than one percent, but these five thousand people die out of the million and five hundred thousand diagnosed. This brings the percentage of victims to the same thirty percent as from the plague.

The horrific numbers are almost forgotten now, just a hundred years after the discovery of antibiotics. From its emergence, to the discovery of a bacterial species that caused the disease, the knowledge that ship rats are the principle cause for the spread of it, and, finally, the notion that hygiene would prevent its return.

> *The Black Death that swept through Europe in the 14th century killed an estimated 25 million people, or 30–60% of the European population. Because the plague killed so many of the working population, wages rose and some historians have seen this as a turning point in European economic development. (Cipolla)*

Churches were built all over Europe to stop the devastation of the plague of 1630. The church of Santa Maria Della Salute was one. The effort succeeded and the plague did subside.

This is Venice.

**DEDICATION &
CERTIFICATION OF
THANKS TO:**

*Vitalia
Golubovskaya*

**ANNA THANKS YOU FOR
YOUR KIND SUPPORT!**

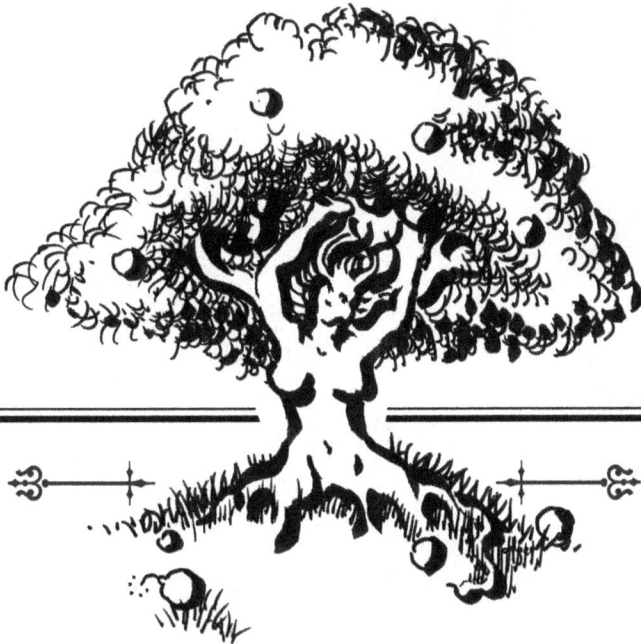

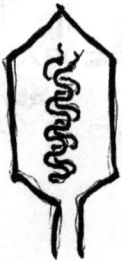

CHAPTER 40

Sodium butyrate

All this time, I was taking Sodium Butyrate on the gentle but insistent demand of Dr. Dmitry. He emailed a set of scientific papers containing references to the roots of Sodium Butyrate's biological action, describing its influence on malignant growth. This was the first of many hundreds of emails we later exchanged when we were developing patents. I skimmed the articles, back then, lacking the time for the level of thinking necessary to truly absorb them. The only thing I managed to grasp was that sodium butyrate operates on chromatin, a ladder of proteins that supports DNA's flexible and thin double helix. I was no stranger to chromatin, because it happened to have been the topic of my Master's thesis: "The influence of Ca, Mg and Na on the compactization of avian erythrocytes' chromatin."

It was defended successfully, but it was hell. My advisor, Dr. Vladimir Semenov, made me build my thesis around his insufficient, monotonous and seemingly indefensible ideas. I had never felt that lost and incompetent in my University career. It was my first encounter with something seemingly legitimate and accepted, but at the same time totally empty.

❈ **I** ❈

Dr. Semenov was one of the very few people in cell biology in The Russian Institute of Cellular Biology who was allowed to go to the West and work at a German bio lab. Of course, he had to be perceived as "safe" for the regime. He was, for instance, not a Jew. He was a very legitimate person, unlike me for example, a half-Jewish girl. His father was a Red Army General... He had an aura of a person who worked with real Western scientists. He was not very imaginative, however, dogmatic and, as I understand now, perhaps just jealous.

I started my work in his lab as an extracurricular activity when I was a third year student of Biochemistry at the Saint Petersburg University's Biology Department. I was not allowed to conduct experiments for the whole first year, when I was confined to washing biological tubes and dishes. Dr. Vladimir had a fervent mendicant, a PhD student named Lesha Petrushkin, with whom I did not get along, to put it mildly. Lesha Petrushkin would inspect every single test tube I washed for spots and turbid areas left by detergent by turning it against the dim Saint Petersburg sun light as it poured through the dirty institutional windows. To reach the point of inspection, the test tubes were soaked for two hours in the deadly "chromka" solution of chromium bisulfate in sulfuric acid. This substance burns biologic matter into atoms of carbon and nitrogen. If it spilled on one's clothes, the result would be disastrous.

Here is the recipe of chromka from the Russian Wikipedia (which, for some cute old world orthodox reason, is called Tradion):

Существует много рецептур этого распространённого лабораторного препарата[1].

- *Состав 1:*
Бихроматкалия – 60 г
Концентрированная серная кислота – 80 мл
Вода – 270 мл

- *Состав 2:*
Бихроматкалия – 15 г
Концентрированная серная кислота – 500 мл

(Composition 1:
Sodium dichromate – 60g
Concentrated sulfuric acid – 80 ml
Water – 270 ml

Composition 2:
Sodium dichromate – 15g
Concentrated sulfuric acid – 500 ml)

During the preparation (adding sulfuric acid to chromium) the vapors of sulfuric acid were visible under the ventilation hood. Sometimes people would cough a bit from the vapors. But work is work, and test tubes had to be clean no matter what vapors had to be inhaled. Here are a few words from Wikipedia:

> **chromic acid** *is usually used for a mixture made by adding concentrated sulfuric acid to a dichromate, which may contain a variety of compounds, including solid chromium trioxide. This kind of chromic acid may be used as a cleaning mixture for glass...This application has declined due to environmental concerns. As with*

*other Cr^{VI} compounds, potassium dichromate is
carcinogenic and should be handled with gloves
and appropriate health and safety protection.
The compound is also corrosive and exposure
may produce severe eye damage or blindness.*[9]
*Human exposure further encompasses impaired
fertility, inheritable genetic damage and harm to
unborn children.*

I did feel forced to neglect of my own health. Everyone did.
We were bullied into weathering any hazard in the name
of science. I did not really believe in it, because all I was
doing was washing test tubes, but I was afraid to admit that
I was doing so badly in life. Some people were luckier. They
had real teachers and they stayed in the labs late at night
and on weekends, but they were producing real results. I,
on the other hand, was assigned someone who was not fit
to teach. He was not kind or generous, but thrifty with his
knowledge, condescending.

❆ II ❆

Chromka splashed on my jeans once or twice and, after a
couple of hours, I noticed a little hole. In a warm room at a
friend's house, I sat down to eat. My jeans had a small hole
in the thigh. An hour later, when I stood up, the hole was so
big that everyone noticed it. They made fun of me: "What
is it? Rapidly growing hole? Wow. A live hole." They had a
moment of revenge. I was the only one whose relatives lived
in the US. Everybody was envious of my American jeans.

They were my very, very prized possession. I looked

extremely Western and extremely cool in my American jeans. I looked like a Western girl, better than the rest of the people on the street. It was a sign of elegant rebellion, a sign that declared: "You can't have me! I am here just by accident! I am a normal Western person, kind and smart, not like these aggressive and primitive types that would cut your throat in a bread line."

I can recall the stories my mother told about her waiting, her life in line. She exchanged her time for sugar, that the state rationed. My reaction was not to stand; not to vie for food; to do something better with my life. Jeans were a sign of being above, of another life, of a better life, where people did not have to stand in lines for food. Jeans in Russia... ogh! This sumptuous subject was cooked into stories about the Soviet Union so many times. Still, it is fresh as an old Beatles' song, beautiful and immortal. A song about love and fighting the system, about being young and rebellious and desiring a non-Soviet slavery life. People were known to pay their entire salaries for a single pair of jeans on the black market. I got mine from my uncle who immigrated to the US and sent them for my birthdays. My jeans were my most cherished possession, the envy of my friends, worn frequently and with pride.

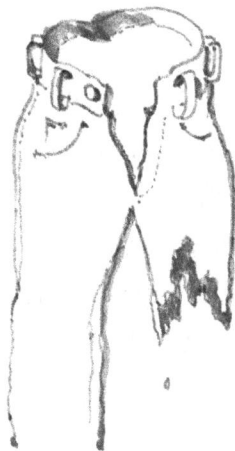

The day the deadly chromka splashed on my jeans, the hole grew steadily. We all watched, wide-eyed. By the end of dinner my thigh was half-naked. I had to rush home because it

was winter and cold to walk like that, and because I did not
know if the hole would continue growing and I would have
no jeans on me at all in a couple of hours. My friend lived
on Liteinyi, and I lived about an hour away on metro in
Veselyi Poselok. In the metro I was trying to cover the hole
inside my coat.

But all my heroic suffering with chromka and washing
test tubes was left unappreciated. I was not ready for the
experiments with avian erythrocyte chromatin, yet. With
sadistic fervor, Lesha Petrushkin continually inspected the
quality of my work for a year and would declare to the boss
it was inadequate. Two hours in chromka. Two detergent
washes. Rinse each test tube ten times with tap water.
Rinse each tube two times with distilled water. Place into a
hot thermostat for at least 2 hours. Cool down. Don't spill
anything. Be perfect.

✁ III ✁

The experiments were planned years in advance and were
performed on a regular basis with very little modification.
One experiment had to do with Ca, another with Mg, one
with concentrations from 10 mg to 100, another from 100
to 1000. It was routine.

The Chromatin Lab kept producing the same
experiments related to the pigeons cooped in an
aviary on the roof of the Institute. It was Lesha
Petrushkin's job to tend to the pigeons. His last name is
avian too, I never thought about it! It means 'a cuckoo.' The
main thing would be the treatment of nuclei, first with Na,

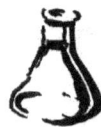

Ca or Mg, then with the enzyme that cuts DNA inside the nuclei, followed by a comparison of two patterns of cutting. Monovalent atoms of Na would be distinguished from bivalent atoms of Ca and Mg. Comparison was done by isolating DNA from the nuclei (avian erythrocyte) and electrophoresis. The electrophoresis required a gel slab which would be prepared by dissolving polyacrylamide powder and leaving the residual solution to polymerize between two glass plates for some time under the red light.

When the solution solidified, the plates with the gel were put into an electrophoresis chamber with a buffer. DNA was loaded into wells on top of the gel slab with a very thin syringe. This was done very precisely so that the precious solution would not leak into a neighboring well or out into the buffer. Then the current was applied. DNA from each of the aliquots would be loaded into a dozen to two dozen wells, depending on the number of samples. DNA would rush to the negative pole, smearing the gel. Since the smallest fragments travel the furthest, the smear would be a function of the size of fragments into which the DNA was cut. Chromatin is the little protein scaffolding blocks that support genetic material inside the nucleus, wrapped around the ladder of nucleosomes. Cutting chromatin with the enzyme exposes genetic material on the surface of the scaffold.

At that point in the procedure, the current would be stopped. The exposed DNA in the gel would be isolated on the glass covering the UV-light lamp in the dark room. The light would be turned off, the cassette of photographic film opened, a piece of film big enough for a few snapshots would be cut. The slightly moist film ribbon would be inserted into the small cassette for the camera, all in the dark. The cassette would be inserted into the camera, the camera would be installed on the frame above the gel, and the UV lamp turned on.

In the UV twilight of the dark room, the DNA spots glistened on the blue glass: pink, beautiful bands of molecules of the same size. Photographs would be snapped at different exposure times and diaphragm widths to get the best depth for a picture, the UV lamp turned off, the film taken out from the cassette and rolled into the small development spool. At this point in the procedure, the light in the dark room could be turned on. The pre-made solution of developing liquid would be poured into the development spool, and the film would be frequently swirled for ten to twenty minutes. The solution went back to the stock solution bucket. The film would be rinsed with water, then rinsed in a stop bath, then into a fixing bath while swirling and finally rinsed one last time with water. Once the film was hung to dry, Dr. Vladimir could see the results.

In the presence of Na, the DNA would be cut at an increment of one nucleosome, in the presence of Ca or Mg, the increment would be two nucleosomes. I was supposed to see bands of the DNA of 130 base pairs, 260 (130X2), 390 (130X3), 520(130X4) in the Na sample, and 260, 520 etc in Ca/Mg. That was all.

My nightmares from then on were of iridescent pink bands of DNA blinking at me under the UV light in the dark room. I did this for two years. Actually three, but the first year I was only permitted to perfect my test-tube washing skills. For my Master's thesis, I had a displayed a number of theses slides to demonstrate a law of single vs double repeat, depending on the metal ion used in a preparation. It was meaningless work I had a feeling would not get me a good grade. I had to incorporate this "data" into the body of science. It was torture, but I did it by reading all about chromatin, active and inactive genes, the conformation of DNA as prepared for transcription. The bulky transcription machinery would not be able to read DNA and RNA by merely moving along the DNA strand. That was why it had to be exposed.

I managed to get an "A," but it was a labor of hate. I never thought I would come back to the problems of chromatin, ever again. Now, with the references to histone deacytylase inhibitors that Dr. Dmitry sent me, I had to go back to the nightmare of chromatin structure. Thirty years after I finished my thesis, I find myself studying the chemicals that modify chromatin condensation. It appears that these chemicals may be a new class of drugs for treating cancer. One of these chemicals is sodium butyrate. I started to take sodium butyrate. Then gradually I read some of the articles Dr. Dmitry sent me.

❊ **IV** ❊

Sodium butyrate and other Histone Deacetylase Inhibitors inhibit the process of holding chromatin so it is inaccessible to the cellular machinery. Acetylation keeps chromatin open. Reading a report like this: "With inhibition of HDAC, histones are acetylated (Ac), and the DNA that is tightly wrapped around a de-acetylated histone core relaxes. We propose that the accumulation of acetylated histones in nucleosomes leads to expression of specific genes, which, in turn, leads to cell growth arrest, differentiation, and/or apoptotic cell death and, as a consequence, an inhibition of tumor growth"

It is clear is that epigenetics is becoming a new industry. When I google epigenetics, I see so many companies producing laboratory kits for studying a gene's epigenetic state. One could order a custom set of genes, or a suggested set of "cancer-related pathways" or "apoptosis pathways." It looks like this knowledge is right around the corner.

But, before we know why sodium butyrate helps, it makes sense to should trust the data we have so far. In the words of the very knowledgeable and very practical Dr. Dmitry: "Why wait to understand what it is that works, if it works?"

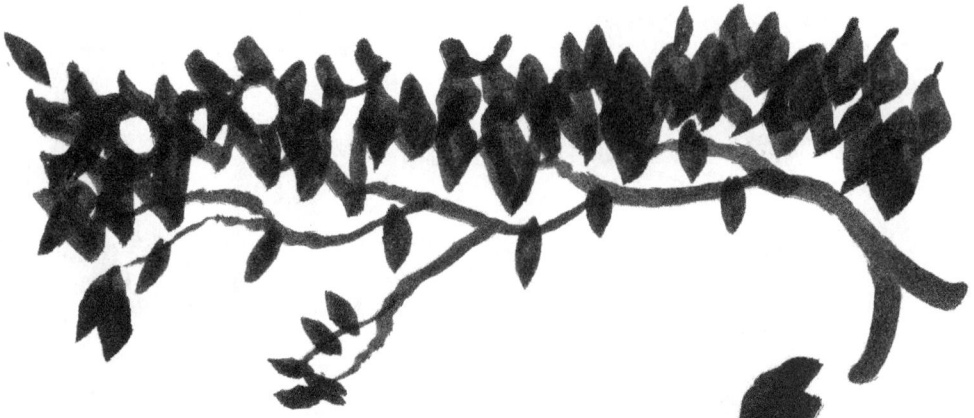

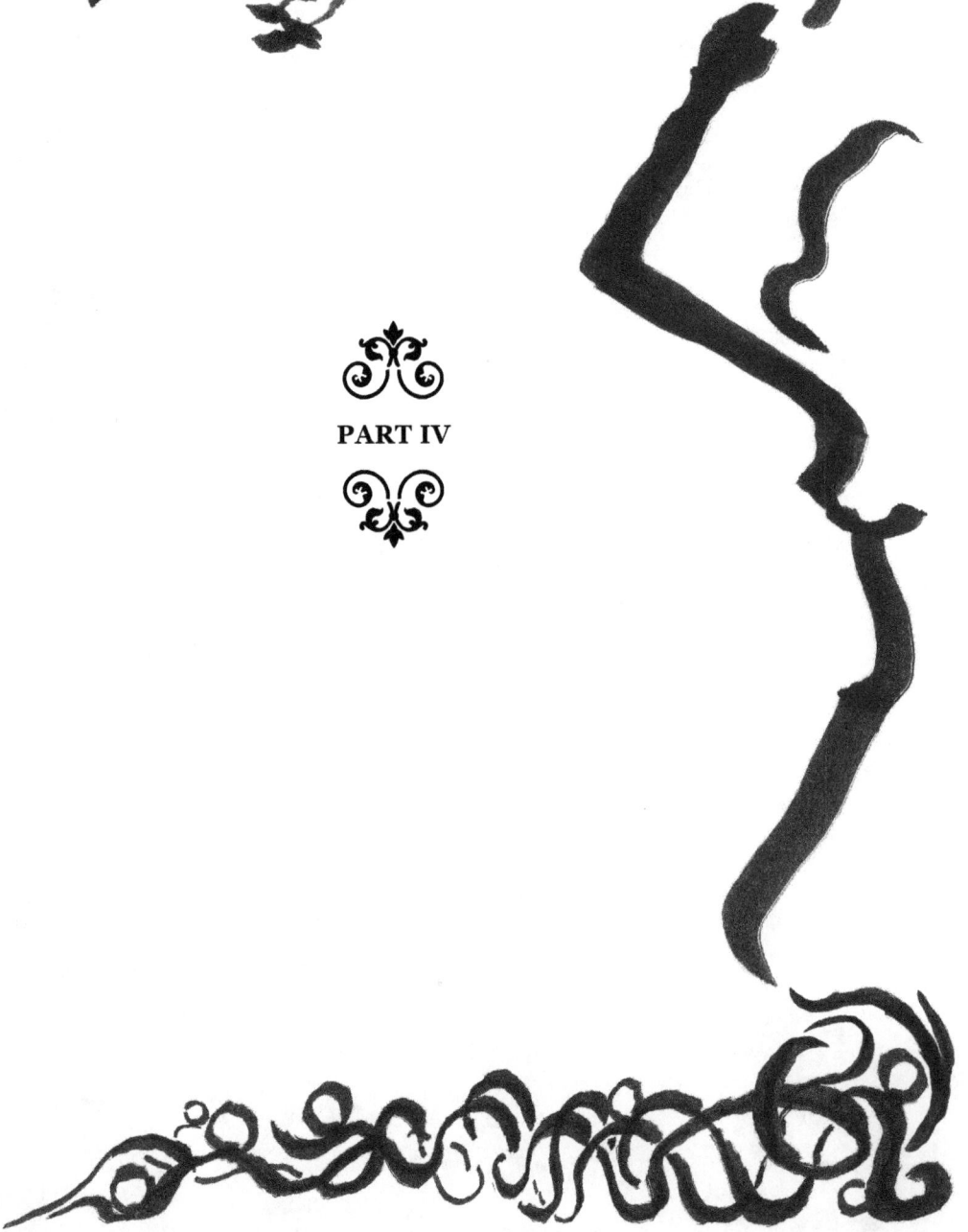

PART IV

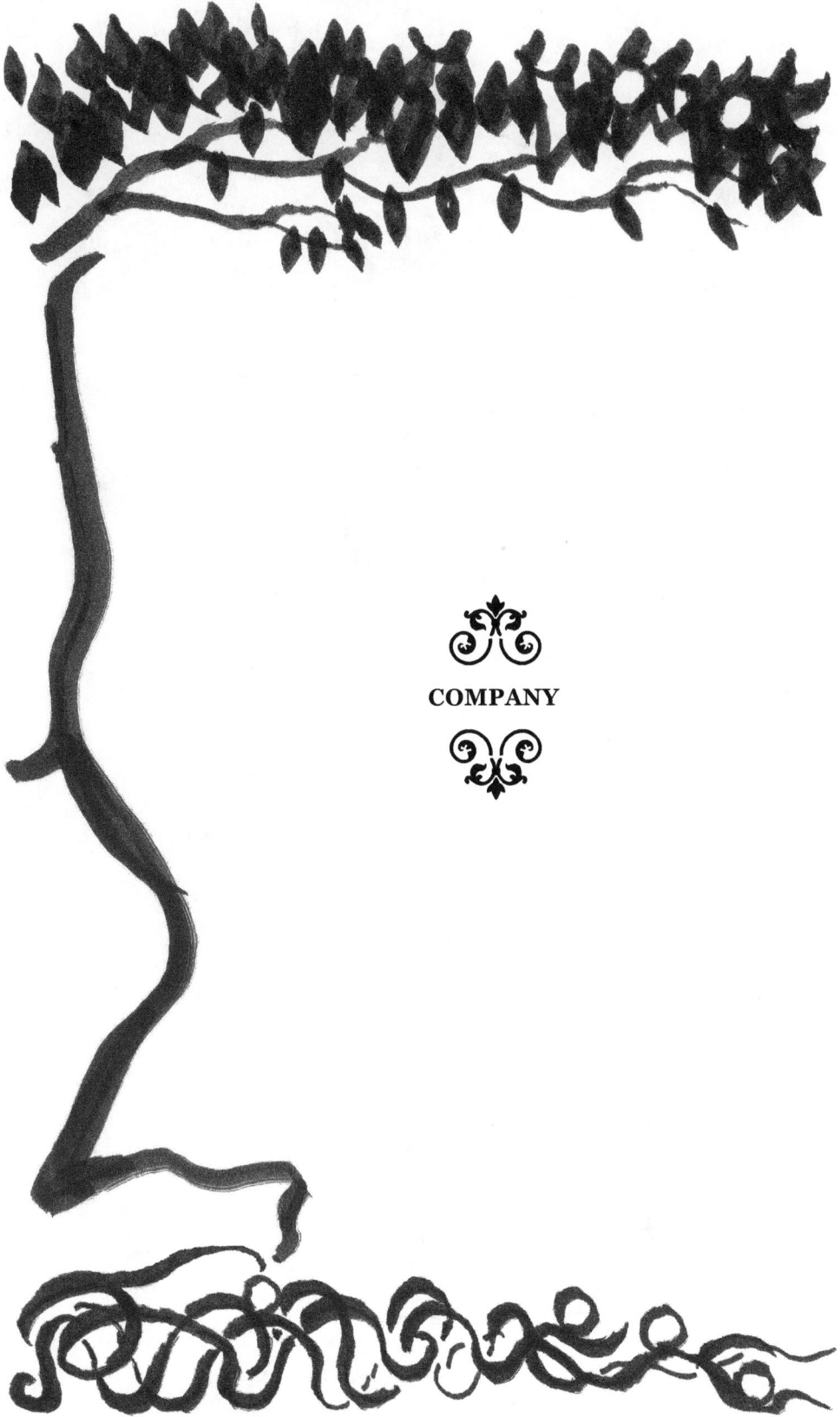

COMPANY

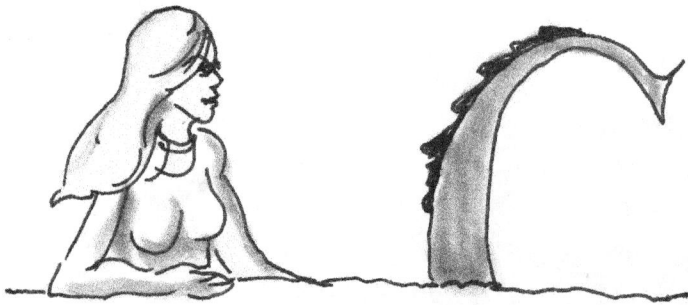

CHAPTER 41

Anna and the Beast

Roll back to the days of desperation and struggles.

Glenn's "How can I help you, Anna?" was a mantra in my life back then. He was an honest friend who did not just grieve about my circumstances and my deadly disease, but who asked relevant questions. His kindness was genuine. He did not ask me for the list of my expenses. He simply said at one point, "Of course I understand that you need a lot of money to do all your treatments." I nodded.

"Would you let me help you?" I nodded again. By that time I gradually opened up to the world. I stopped being ashamed of my cancer. Glenn suggested I get my friends together to help out with the money for getting well. At first, of course, I was not sure how much I would want to let everyone know. I was still so afraid of being reviled or pitied. One of my college friends stopped talking to me when she found out I had cancer. She wanted to keep focused on positivity. I didn't blame her or anyone else for their reactions, and didn't want to subject them to discomfort, especially in the name of asking for help. I looked inside. Lance Armstrong was already there with his detailed and honest account of his treatments, fears and money worries. Annette was already there with her bald head at the local supermarket. The shame of having cancer was not totally gone, but was diminished just enough for me to give Glenn a list of the emails of everyone I considered a friend.

So, one day, Glenn wrote an email to all those of my dear friends that I included on the list. Most of them already knew I had cancer. It was such a joy to see their enthusiasm and desire to help out! There were several meetings at Lena and Mark's house and it was a good time together. Their house is so often the scene of warm parties and heated intellectual conversations. My witty and clever friends came up with the plan: to have a fundraiser with an art twist. Drinking, eating and laughing, we came up with a plan to do a web site. Would it be .org or .net? What is the name? My daughter, Naomi, had written a book about a princess, wrestling a beast. Mark made a little project out of her book several years ago. It came up now. "Bingo!" Greg said, "Anna and the Beast!" The name for the website was born.

Several people did the web site: Mark and Curt as designers, Iden as a wordpress expert and the main programmer, Gosha as a helping hand, Glenn as the CEO of the whole operation. I want to thank you all, and of course you too, Friederike. I'd like to thank Lena, for providing her house and thoughts and, later, her beautiful art work for the auction. I'd like to thank Alex Seltzer for going around the neighborhood asking for support. And you too, Vicki, for your common sense. And you too, Connie, for your faith in me and for your fundraising among local businesses. Thank you, Lynn, for your business sense. And you too, and you too, all my dear friends. Some of the people on my list that were handed over to Glenn were the members of La Salle University Women's MBAs organization. They too became part of the effort, very active and efficient. I would love to thank you too, June, for organizing my La Salle women MBAs friends, and you too Liz, Sharmell Marie and Adelle for designing and selling "Anna and the Beast" t-shirts at the fund raiser, and you too, Latoya Marie and Terry for your ongoing encouragement and faith in me.

Iden, you put many hours to get the web site (annaandthe-beast.org) up and running. Mark, your designs were beautiful. Mark created an old Russian Book of Psalms out of our family photos and bits of my texts. The web site was made in a couple of weeks, and some people donated money this way. I thank you all here again. If not for your support, I might not be here now.

The next thing they planned was the art auction. At this auction, my artist friends sold their works and donated the money to my treatments. I also sold a couple of my own photographs of Saint Petersburg that Mark had suggested we print. How exciting! Thank you Mark and Lena, you donated most of the works. Thank you, all who bought them.

I've wanted to thank you all for so long. I am so glad to be doing this now.

At the fundraiser, Naomi sang a song: "What a wonderful world." Ten years old, she played her guitar and she sang so beautifully that many people in the audience cried. Thank you, darling. It was a beautiful gathering at the Abington Friends School to which a lot of parents of Simon and Naomi's former classmates came. This event was a moving celebration. I made a short, funny speech to make the whole event a little bit less solemn. Joking was my way of keeping myself from crying. There were many reasons to be joyful, with so many people coming to support me and my family.

Ten thousand dollars were made at this fundraiser. That gave me peace of mind for a while and allowed me to travel to Russia freely and pay for treatments without the backdrop of worries about money. That was a freedom I had never experienced before. What an unbelievable gift from Glenn, from all my friends, and from all those perfect strangers who rushed to help.

DEDICATION & CERTIFICATION OF THANKS TO:

The members of Jenkintown International Friends with special gratitude to Carrie Goldhill and Sayda Lam

ANNA THANKS YOU FOR YOUR KIND SUPPORT!

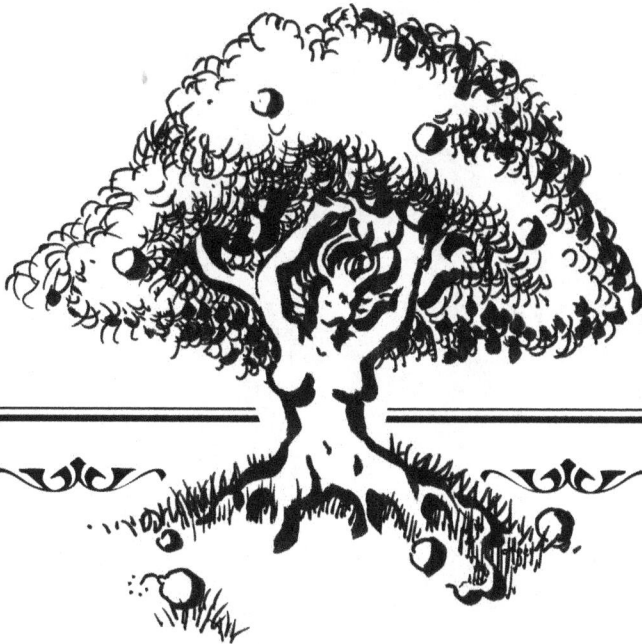

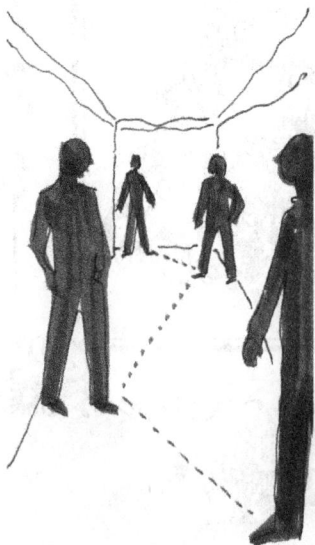

CHAPTER 42

Airports

My life was saved by Russian scientists, this is forever. Russian scientists. From mother Russia. But I hate the Moscow airport. It's like one big inner argument between Russian conservatives, Russian liberals, Russian pro-government, Russian anti-Putin, Russian pro-Orthodox Church's statehood, Russians for separation of church and state, Russian poets, Russian oligarchs, and the Russian middle class. Sheremetyevo-2 is an extremely unfriendly place for any human being. The Moscow airport is hostile and dirty and, if you say so, they accuse you of being anti-Russian. So, I tried to avoid it. The airport, that is.

— I —

After years of subjecting themselves to the advice of the West, Russia is allergic to criticism on all levels. They are especially hostile to visiting ex-pats. A Russian scientist saved my life. I am tremendously grateful to him; he is my third parent.(However I have at least four. Or wait. I have many, lesser of a parent than him but still, kind of sub-parents, who contributed to my vaccine.) But he is the main second-tier parent. I am from Russia. I was born in the center of its Universe, in Leningrad, on Goncharnaya Street, near the Moscow Station: a railroad that connects the two famous cities of Moscow and Saint Petersburg.

When I was still a little girl, my family moved into a "new flat" – a Soviet cinder block apartment on the outskirts of Saint Petersburg that was built as part of the economic plan. I loved my old city neighborhood, but I hated the new one. There was nothing around the buildings. Fields of dirt, emptied villages. I hated this anti-utopia naked landscape around. However the flat was spacious and light. My new village-born, street-smart neighbors showed me very early the darker side of Russia. Their parents were forced to leave the villages devastated by the Soviet state and come to the city to work in factories. The factories were semi-dilapidated, pre-revolutionary buildings brought out of retirement to meet the production quotas of the Five Year Communist Party Plan (Piatiletka). My neighbors filled buses and trolleys every morning to get to the factories, which were located an hour away. Every evening, they filled the same buses home, lined up near the many beer booths to get drunk and went home to get yelled at by their suffering wives.

Many of these people were chronic alcoholics. God knows how they functioned: shadows of people, barely registering life around them. Their children quickly organized into gangs that targeted "urbanites." In my local school, I was once attacked by a pack of boys: lining the narrow hall, they terrorized me by pushing me in a zig-zag pattern from boy to boy, each one holding his dirty hand over my mouth to keep me from screaming. They knew all kinds of street-smart tricks. Sadly, most of them died or went to prison before making any mark on the world. One girl from my apartment complex became a prostitute when she was very young. The street became off limits to me, because these gangs were vengeful and merciless. I did not tell my parents about the incident in the hallway because I was afraid they would start an investigation. I did beg them to transfer me to another school and, somehow, through my father's connections, succeeded in sending me to a different district.

Every day, I would take a bus packed with factory workers. The crowd was thick, and had to force myself into the bus and out at my school stop. The workers continued on on the bus to their factories for another 20 minutes. At school, I appeared a little shaky from the morning bus travel and breathing in the worker's yesterday spirit. Perhaps some times I prayed to leave that place as soon as possible, even though I could not even dream of it. Each of us was heavily depressed and scared of each other and of the state. The villagers and their kids, the urbanites and their kids, the teachers who taught both, the bus drivers: we were all afraid.

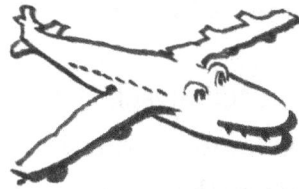

The only cheerful bunch were the shop clerks. They were dismissive and aloof, kissed-up to by hungry masses, fearless in their re-distribution dealings. They toyed with the officials who could jail them for the multiple mini-crimes they committed every day. They despised the average folk for lacking the guts to cross the line of the inadequate law and create their own happiness. In the 70's and 80's, these masters of their own destiny became the heroes of songs by Vysotsky and then, with a more criminalized flavor, the songs of Rosenbaum. These songs foreshadowed the future Darwinian struggles that rolled out in Russia in the brutal and bloody 90's. By then, I was trying to make it in America.

← II →

It would be tempting and "Russian" of me to say that it's love that gives one the right to criticize. It would be a nice cliché. But, in America, I learned something else: those with insight have a responsibility to voice it. So, I am far from bashing Russia when I say that the Moscow airport was definitely something to avoid at all costs. My mind would fill with turmoil every time I stepped onto Moscow soil and ungratefully felt annoyed by its hostility and the squeamishness of the service people at the airport. The products of a cold and hostile nature and centuries of social Darwinism, these new species of people had to be forgiven for being what they were. At times, I would wonder if Russia's resilience and stubbornness were necessary elements in creating my dendritic vaccine.

I amused myself that Peter the Great did something similar to what many Russians did after him: he went to the West to learn the Western way of life. He realized that experiencing, first hand, how other nations lived was the key to a fantastic positive change. Not only did he send a lot of Russians to study abroad, he invited foreigners to come to Russia and build, develop, create, live. Saint Petersburg was built by Italian architects. Germans came to develop science and manufacturing, and the French were the strongest influence on literature and politics. This was always a topic for many lofty discussions.

I had a conversation with my Russian lawyer, who was very interested in why I left Russia. I heard this question many times from Americans, and I learned how to match my answer to my audience. But I never, ever heard it from a

Russian. My friends never questioned my desire to live in a different country, to have a different perspective, a different life. I am very blessed that no one ever asked. It showed a respect for my privacy. But, when my lawyer asked, I had to look into myself and address his implied criticism of my negligence towards my country.

Good people who decided to stay definitely had a special aura. In the struggle of good and evil that followed the end of the Soviet Union, they represented soldiers of good standing against all wild evil turned up by the social turmoil, namely the Bloody Nineties. Gosha and I sympathized with the struggles of Russian people. Sometimes we would even take the blame: "if we did not leave Russia, it would have been a better country." Guilt is a Russian's favorite feeling. So I told my curious lawyer, "It does not matter why I left, but look at me as an asset now. I have traveled to the other end of the world. Use me now. Russia, use me now."

I know what he was thinking: You were there while we suffered here. Everything that happened to Russia became my fault also because I dared to choose a different life. This is a frequent sentiment. But now I am back begging for help and had to take responsibility for being so shallow. In Russia everybody thinks along the lines of polarization.

I was almost looked at as an enemy. The definition of enemy would be somebody who did not share their horrific experience with them. There is no resolution for me in sight unless I become as great as Dr. Dmitry, working my heart away for mankind.

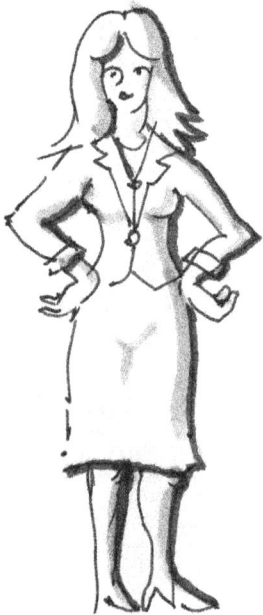

CHAPTER 43

Startup

Before I got sick, I started to get involved in the
Philadelphia startup scene. My favorite organization is the
Philadelphia Startup Leaders. When I joined them, they
were some young tech guys, who had been getting together
at local bars for about a year to throw around ideas. It
grew so much in four years that it is now a very diverse and
rather formal organization with a president and a structure.
But they still meet at the bars, and there would be people
who would listen to any wild ideas anyone can think of
making into a business, and there are very successful companies that were started in Philly bars.

I was not as young and as tech-savvy, but the scene was
inspiring. With no boundaries around what they could
conceive and sometimes selling their companies or licenses
for millions of dollars, it just seemed like a perfectly
successful life. I was hooked forever. It was clear to me that
there would always be enough laughter, knowledge and
friendly advice to support my efforts.

When I realized my 6 month prognosis had long passed
and I was still alive, I decided to start a business. I wanted
to make a living for myself saving lives and I wanted to
make Dr. Dmitry rich. I knew he was scrambling for money.
His vaccine was a miracle the world should know about. It
seemed like a dormant seed. I realized how easy it would be
to develop Dr. Dmitry's technologies in the US, how many
more people would be cured, how much more money could

be made, and just how beautiful it would be. It could be a new life for Dr. Dmitry, if he wanted it. "Let's try," he said, "I don't really believe in all of these dreams of yours, Anya, but I could have an American patent on my wall: that alone would be enough." I was very very excited.

"Oh and by the way," Dr. Dmitry said in passing, "There is an investor. I cured him from Big Infectious C. Talk to him."

Even more excited, I rolled up my sleeves.

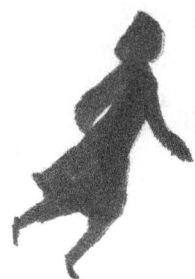

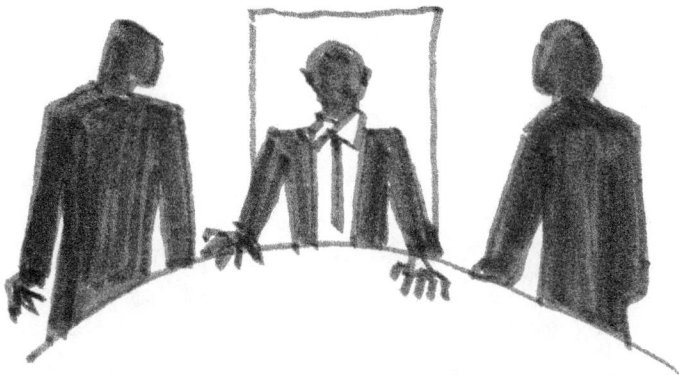

CHAPTER 44

The First Meeting

We agreed to meet with the investor at a strange café, in a small street right off Saint Petersburg's main drag, Nevsky Prospect. The café was rather shabby and reminded me of the Soviet era "stolovaya" with a traditional menu of mashed potatoes, a pickle and meatloaf in gravy. It would usually be accompanied by "compote," the remnant of French cuisine in pre-revolutionary Russia. Most the cafes in Saint Petersburg are very modern and quite upscale. The investor called and announced he was running late.

"Okay," I said. "No problem." I took it as a declaration of dominance; from the outset he wanted to create a clear hierarchy. So I had to sit there alone and smell the cheap Soviet era meatballs with gravy and mashed potatoes.

I ordered green tea. I was in a good mood, as I always was these days. I knew I looked good in my wig and my totally foreign and unusually modest for a Russian taste American clothing. Different is always good. The investor arrived with a girl, obviously his girlfriend. In the Russian tradition, she was at least twenty years younger.

"Cyrill."

"Anna."

Cyrill Rotkov was a slender man in jeans and a sweater. I have seen investors before. This one seemed nice and friendly but, moreover, he was recommended by Dr. Dmitry so he was "in." The girlfriend took a very active part in the discussion. She often interrupted his slow, importantly paused speech. She was smart and reasonable. We talked about his interest in Big Infectious C and my interest in cancer. He told me how he was cured from Big Infectious C, how he almost died, and how nobody was able to help. I told him about my cancer and how I had delayed the death sentence by six months, already.

"You understand this is something nobody would let us do?" he said, speaking of the patent I proposed.

"No. Not really."

"Well, you are very naïve."

"Why?"

"Because this is like an oil well. You can't come to it with a bucket."

"What bucket? Why not?"

"Seriously, you're that naïve? The big boys will not let you."

"You can sell the company to the big boys..."

"My friend was killed in a car accident. We worked together."

"Sorry."

"You still don't understand."

"He died. I am sorry."

"Killed."

"Oh?!"

"Yeah."

I was really puzzled where he was going.

"Big boys?!" I inferred.

"You bet. Now you are getting it!"

"Oh no."

"Yeah."

I was processing what he was saying. He hinted that the big "boys" were vicious Big Pharma. My American point of view was different. I believed that company development could be done in a civilized way.

"We can develop it and work with them, with lawyers..."

I almost saw a shadow of the Russian Wild And Bloody Nineties looming over the conversation. The shadow was still smoking with a deadly danger. How can I even try to describe the Bloody Nineties! I was not there. But when silence falls in the middle of a discussion, this is the reminder of that dark period in Russia's recent history. Perhaps the survivors reminisce about their fallen friends, or about the immoral choices they had to make at the gunpoint of a liberated thug, or about the people who were killed because an uncontrolled criminal mind decided to obtain their assets, offices, money, and cars.

It was all about how far a criminal mind could go without the restriction of a functioning society. And they went far. The city was flooded with gangs. Gangs seemed to be the only standing order in a society that suddenly crumbled from its false ideological foundation. It was total chaos. Nothing stood. Nothing remained. Only human nature in its very basic Darwinian form. My scientist friends reported going hungry. They were not paid salaries. The scientific institutions did not have money for heating bills and rented out the labs to anyone with a little bit of money. Today, the Bloody Nineties, is the painful past that everybody tries to forget in order to move on as a society. But the skills of that Darwinian era made people's character. Utmost suspicion, lying, aggression, and taking sides in deeply polarized society make up the norm in people's interatctions.

I indeed was from another planet.

"Do you understand where I am heading, or you are going to continue to play naïve?!"

That was a little bit too harsh. I stared at him and his girlfriend. Then, the moment of embarrassment passed, and the girlfriend enthusiastically started to say something about organizing patients in groups for the fight for a cure. My enthusiasm was absolute, so that no moments of silence and embarrassment could have affected it. I instantly switched to a positive conversation again.

"Great idea!"

She chirped something smart, again.

"Great idea." I kept repeating.

I tried to keep the conversation friendly, with my best intentions.

"We could do a lot of things together. In the US I am connected with a start-up community... With women's organizations..."

"Hmm. That's a good idea. All of those powerful women together, sharing things between themselves."

"We can do it in many ways. We just need to start working on a plan," I said.

"I was here in the 90's, you weren't. You know nothing, my friend," he said.

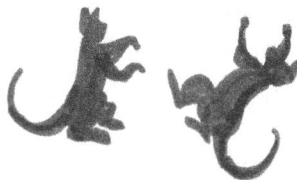

With this we said a rather friendly goodbye to each other and left the café.

Being absent from Russia in the 90's, I did not witness the rise of the primal Darwinian morale. Gradually, I reconstructed the picture of the Russian society where the domination of the alpha-males was an obligatory ritualistic spectacle: a Greek tragedy with spectators, a chorus, and a hero. He makes his demise or victory a public event, an eternal play where he is the actor and all else are spectators. He feels he is always watched, always fighting, and that he must prove himself.

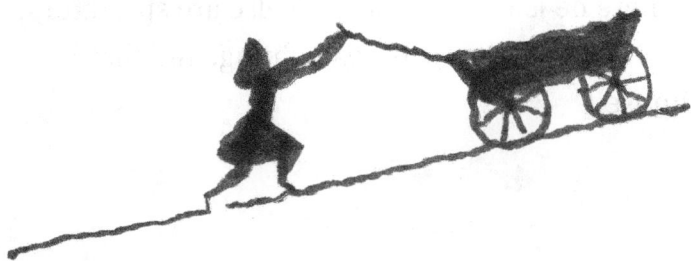

CHAPTER 45

Agreement

⋗ I ⋖

Ivan Ivanych, my Russian business mentor, a self-de-scribed social-good entrepreneur, is quite famous in Saint Petersburg circles. He agreed to guide me through the beginning of a business. I had just finished my chemo. It was October of 2009. I knew nothing about intellectual property law, but Iv Iv used to work with a lawyer and IP counselor he recommended. He set up an appointment for me and I went to meet my first of many lawyers.

Maxim Kluglov was a former chemist. He had a nice new office in what looked like a regular flat in a quiet old Petersburg inner courtyard. I came to him, excited about the road ahead. I was excited all the time, those days. Iv Iv accompanied me for the first introductory meeting. We took off our shoes in the foyer and put on house slippers. It felt so much like home.

"Tea or coffee?"

We sat on an Italian leather sofa, Maxim sat at the table. They chatted about Maxim's son, and his wife, his summer vacation, and his paintings. Ivan Ivanych went into a long discussion about the quality of the paintings. Maxim was glancing at his wrist watch. Slowly, Ivan Ivanych came to the point, the reason for our visit.

"OK," Maxim said. "Immunotherapy? No problem. Let's

keep in touch via email."

"Just send him a letter asking for his rates," Ivan said to me.

I exchanged cards with Maxim. He listed his achievements: "I am a rather expensive lawyer. And I am a busy one. I don't insist that you hire me."

This trick always works on me. We met again in his office in couple of days, this time Ivan did not accompany me.

"Don't even start without an agreement," he insisted.

"What do you mean? I trust them completely. Dr. Dmitry saved my life."

"Things happen, especially with investors. I've seen it happen multiple times."

"How?"

"Naïve people like you will work on something and then your so-called investor will come in and say 'Thank you for the good work, you may leave now. And they will just take the whole thing and push the poor inventor out.'"

"Why do you think this might happen to me?" It seemed all so unlikely. I felt like me, Dr. Dmitry and Cyrill were already a team put together in heaven.

"I am not saying they will. I am just saying they might. They probably will... I know they will... They always do!"

Maxim was a quiet man, with the soft manners of a cat.

But by the end of this phrase he was flashing and agitated, almost yelling.

"I am telling you! I am not doing any patenting work! Before. You. Bring. Me. An. Agreement!"

I sat back in the Italian leather arm chair and the slippers.

"Okay, okay," I said. "I will bring you an agreement."

"It's not for me. It's for you."

"Sure. Thank you."

"It has to say who is doing what. I will help you finalize it as soon as you send me the draft. Just simple and clear, and I will do the rest. Then you will all sign it. Then you will all agree that I represent you."

So, I went to work. Dr. Dmitry and Cyrill had different perspectives on why we were doing what we were doing. What are we doing? I was going back and forth between the two of them. Cyrill said,"I don't care. I just want to cure people. I was cured. And I want to cure people." He looked stern and heroic in these moments. When he was telling me "I almost died," he seemed to be on the brink of tears and at the same time his suffering seemed to give him some kind of moral authority. It works especially well with naïve and compassionate people. I would have submitted to the power of his heroic struggles if I had not been able to reply,"I almost died as well. I am still undergoing chemo."

"But I almost died."

"But me too. Then what?"

"OK never mind, you heard me."

Was he trying to boss me,
or did it just seem that way?
I dismissed all negative
thoughts. My Russian men-
tor, Iv Iv always came up
with the same imperative:
"Whatever. Just keep push-
ing this cart up the hill. Just keep pushing. What's next?"
My questions about implementation were met with a sad
expression on Cyrill's rather classy elongated face, with its
long narrow nose.

"It does not matter. I just want to take it into the clinic." I
could see the pain in his big eyes.

"But how are you going to do it?" I asked.

"You do it. I don't care," and he disappeared into his
beautiful suffering among the streets and alleys of Saint
Petersburg.

I did not know it, back then, but I was already appointed as
the enemy. Cyrill was just waiting for a convenient moment
to find some flaw, or stage a disagreement. His measured
silences were a close study of my potential weaknesses. A
skilled fighter knows this principle: Don't use your own
energy. Use your enemy's energy. Pretend you are with
him, pretend you are him. This will give you a better chance
to strike when he is not anticipating. Appear weak and

distracted. He was getting ready for battle, not for collaboration. He learned business in the Russian 90's. He only knew how to kill an enemy, not how to work together. I did not understand what that meant, back then.

The Russian government is conveniently anti-American. "Everything Microsoft built is based on Russian ideas. And where is the money?!" I've heard this rhetoric from many. It was an easy task to start blaming me for having sympathies towards American lawyers who only wait to take a Russian scientist's ideas and sell them to Big Pharma. It took me many months to awaken from my blind excitement to see the bitter truth of the real game Cyrill was playing.

⚞ II ⚟

Being the judge in waiting, Dr. Dmitry was simply practical.

"I just want to get money for my research."

He at that moment perhaps already knew that Cyrill was not going to let me drive but was pretending and waiting.

"Okay, understood."

"If you just get me an American patent, that would be it. Great."

"Hmm. I think we could do more." I said.

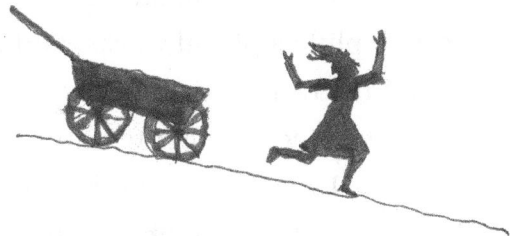

"I just need the American patent. It's important for me to have it on the wall. People react to American credentials but don't react on Russian ones. Anything American supports my reputation."

It is a paradox that in a society where the word "American" is the official propaganda's synonym to "evil," many people spin this propaganda trick to their advantage when they need to. It has a stamp of coolness and superior quality. Russians see everybody as friends or enemies. There are no passersby, no artists, no scientists, no businessmen, no investors, no collaborators, no teachers, no strangers. Only liberals, conservatives, Orthodox, Catholics any delineation that could be divided into fighting camps.

Lenin was a master of finding enemies; the tsar was the enemy, his friends were enemies—spiteful, ugly, camouflaging cowards—and on and on and on. We, the children of the Soviet Union, had to read too much of his hateful, so called philosophical works, and undoubtedly absorbed this hateful attitude towards everybody, towards life. However, he was associated not with the ultimate failure but with victory. Lenin was as passionate as Hitler, and imagine what would have happened to the Germans if they were taught in schools to follow and adore Hitler well after his death. In Russia, they were. Stalin, a seminarian in his youth, perverted the primitive emotions of a jealous man to a Byzantine sophistication.

This is how we grew up: searching for enemies in our closest allies, finding them as soon as we thought we could win the battle that would ensue. Just by virtue of travel, I did not breathe the toxic air as much as many of my dear friends and dear foes did. I was a Russian for twenty eight years and then I was non-Russian for twenty. Sometimes I catch myself searching for those familiar, comforting polarizing dichotomies. Then I stop. I busy myself with real things, like building companies.

I created a draft of the basic agreement and gave it to Maxim. He turned it into a legal document with all the necessary provisions. Then, in March, about six months after we made the decision to build a company, the agreement was signed. The tasks were to be divided as follows: funding was to be provided by Cyrill, technology by Dr. Dmitry, and project coordination by myself.

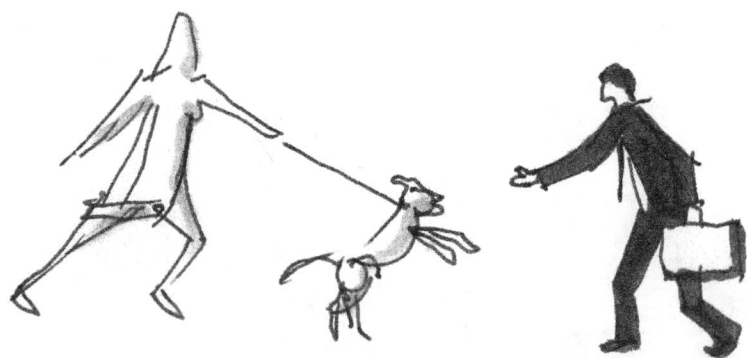

CHAPTER 46
Lawyers and Lawyers

My shrink says I hire so many lawyers because I want someone to be my pit bull. "And then you are disappointed when they turn around and bite you," he says. I agree, I do a lot of business with lawyers. I believe things should be done properly.

❧ I ❧

"Anya, why do you need these documents, these expensive lawyers?" Dr. Dmitry would often say this in a way that sort of meant to show me how irrelevant my activity was. I spent many hours on the phone with Dr. Dmitry, explaining to him why IP was necessary. Dr. Dmitry was visibly fatigued from going over and over this "business" stuff. It clearly took away the precious hours in his lab that he wanted to have for his dialogue with God. I felt sorry for him, and tried to require as little of him as possible.

Cyrill would be silent for weeks. When he did talk, words lost their memory: they meant something one day, and the opposite the next.

"Why did you do that?"

"Because we agreed to."

"No, this is all wrong. You are very difficult to talk to, you know."

I felt like I was sent to buy the cigarettes, I would run to get them, buy the best, and when I would return as a girl sent out to buy cigarettes, panting, returning to her masters, they would scream:

"What have you done!!!"

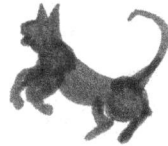

"What?"

"We sent you to buy us vodka. Ha haha," they would laugh. "Did you see what she did, this woman?"

I ended up paying my own money for the cigarettes too. "Get out, and by the way, leave the cigarettes, if you want to stay alive." That's what it was like. It was devilish. The only thing left was fear: Dr. Dmitry was clearly fearful of Cyrill. "He survived the 90's," Dr. Dmitry would say, "he is very tough because of his business." And Dr. Dmitry would smile at me as if he hinted at something awful.

"Bear on," my ethical Russian business mentor, Iv Iv, would say. "Swallow the crap and continue to move this thing forward. If you jump off now, nothing will get done. They won't do a thing. I know this type. This is why you need everything in writing," he would say.

I would continue to work out the plan, in unreliable words. Iv Iv described his work with Maxim as a constant push to get things done. "I would call his office every day and ask detailed questions. That was the only way," he said. When we were writing the patent with Maxim, this process was happening remotely, but I had to prod him daily to keep the patent application moving forward. "Pushing is your job," Iv Iv encouraged me. "Push."

At the end of the day, Dr. Dmitry had cured people, he had patentable protocols, he had the satisfaction of his dialogue with God. I just had a bunch of emails and conversations to follow up on. I was horrified when I realized this. Time had such value for me after my prognosis. I hated doing something so non-tangible, even if it was in the name of building a company.

&8 **II** 8&

The servelist of PSL reads like a book of questions you were always afraid to ask. These young tech guys are fearless and cool. When I posted my question: "Who knows a good lawyer?" I received a lot of heartfelt recommendations and warm advice on how each would be good. This community is really rooting for the success of its members.

I must admit I felt too "Russian" for them: too secretive, too frightened that my ideas could be stolen. It is on every business person's mind and should be. Every entrepreneur learns to maintain an equilibrium regarding what can be shared, and what must be protected. But, in PSL, resources were shared openly and full-heartedly, and with the desire to see others succeed.

The first person to respond to my plea for a lawyer was Mike Righty. We had a phone call very soon after the email and he painted a picture of the road ahead for me. He made everything seem so light and reachable, having had a great deal of startup success. He never pushed, never hurried, never insisted. I aspire to be like that, I can't imagine how he does it. At the time, he had just left a big law firm,

Foerster Hadley Krupp, to start his own one-person firm.
Now his firm has grown to several partners and has offices
in New York City. Go Mike! He held my hand and introduced me to the best startup lawyers in town.

Actually, just lately, his was named the best law firm for
startups. Mike's light approach to doing things is very
winning. I aspire to be like that. I bet if he met with
resistance, Mike would just leave the situation, altogether.
He understands that the world is big and that he should
spend his time with people he can work with. Mike is a
true communicator, in contrast to my collaborators in
Russia. When I shared a strategy or business plan with
my partners, they would respond with a gloomy silence.
Sometimes Cyrill would leave the meeting, citing some
urgent involvements. My enthusiasm was met with
suspicion and silence.

"What I am suspected of?"

"Working for American lawyers. They will snatch
our secrets."

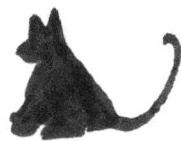

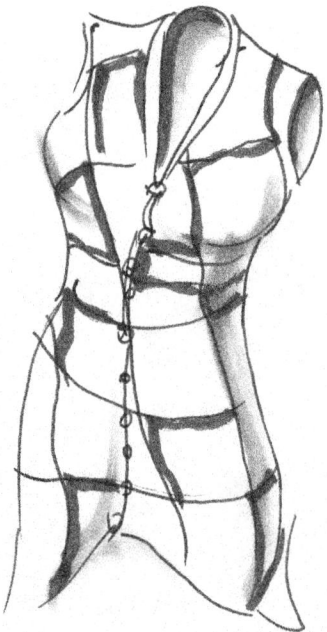

Savonlinna

Citizens of Saint Petersburg try to go produce shopping in
Finland several times a year. The produce is natural there,
while the Russian stores carry fruit and vegetables poisoned
with pesticides and always of the lowest quality. My dear
friend Olga Kotlovaya, a real opera aficionado, went to
Finland for a summer opera festival every year. This summer, she invited me and we went together. Olga showed me
some of the best places I have ever seen adding a fascinating running commentary. On a trip to New York, once, she
showed me several fantastic, fabulous, breath-taking places
by her favorite designer Philippe Starck.

₴ I 3

Olga was an important friend, an active participant in the
recovery of my soul; thoughtful and attentive to the details
and travails of my life, she was always on my side. Olia,
thank you so much! This is my tribute to you! Her witty
professional commentary was an education into design
and aesthetics. I trust her fully. Some years ago, when she
lived and worked in New York, Olga designed our house
in Pennsylvania. It was a great project, for which I had to
educate myself as a client by reading Vladimir Nabokov's
rather obscure novel "Ada." The novel is about a closely knit
family who had to emigrate from one imaginary country
(easily recognizable as Russia) to another imaginary
country (America). Nabokov filled the novel with furs,

diamonds, dance parties, cars and other prohibition era accoutrements: the era of Art Deco, missed by Russia, where the stupid revolution wiped out the furs, the diamonds, the beautiful women with their thin cigarettes and champagne goblets, interesting men, love, and romance.

Very few people have read Ada, but my neighbor, the German-born mathematician Dr. Luther, has an entire bookshelf dedicated to this novel. It includes translations in French, German and English. Dr. Luther is a very private person, so I could not get out of him just why he was so extraordinarily fascinated by this novel. It made him fascinating to me.

Our house redesign project was a protest against the Bloody Revolution and the deprivation it brought to the wealth, the intellect, the soul of those Russians (our great-grand parents) who decided to stay. The infamous project "The zigzag of Ada and Art Deco" was the coolest one that year in the Designer House Tour. This was not as important to me as the process of doing it with Olga, or rather, of watching her do it.

❦ II ❧

Olia took me to Savonlinna, and off we went from the summer of Saint Petersburg to the summer of the Finnish country side. But before that, we stayed in Helsinki for a couple days and did some shopping. We shopped for a dress for me to wear as representative of the company. The dress she chose for me had big black and off-white checkers. It's had a very classic cut, kind of from the 60's, but with a bit of an exaggeration due to the checkers. This was to be my business suit for the summer.

In Savonlinna we met with a wonderful person, Ilpo, who spent a day with us and illuminated Finland for us with stories about his family and his childhood in a village near Savonlinna. His father was a priest, and they lived outside his parish on the lake in a priest's quarters. His mother was the first Finnish woman who attended Finland's School of Architecture, even though her parents were peasants in Karelia. Uneducated themselves but working hard on their farm and saving money so their children could go to school, the whole family in the generation brought up their kids in the spirit of culture and devotion to education, music and architecture. His cousin is a very famous composer. Ilpo, himself, is an opera singer by training and now also a computer scientist. He sang an aria for us in his car. I have to ask Olga if she remembers which one.

The history of this typical Finnish family's road to culture is amazing. They had very difficult lives, these farmers from Karelia. In 1939, they were forced to leave everything behind and move North to an area of Finland that was not occupied and annexed by the Soviets. I did not tell Ilpo that we rented a room every summer in Karelia, near the highway, the Helsinki-Saint Petersburg highway. What if we were living in his family home? I felt guilty living there. From time to time, a beautiful bus carrying Finnish "tourists" would stop by and its passengers would stare at us, children of the occupiers living in now dilapidated houses. Fifty years after they left, their orchards were still producing apples and berries. Half-attended by miserable "occupiers" they were a living, yet bleak memory of a past happiness.

Finland had been part of Sweden, then part of Russia. After it became independent in 1917 as the result of the Revolution, Finland became a fantastic country full of friendly people, educated, prosperous, and environmentally conscious. Such a contrast to my country: a land of toothless, coughing vagabonds hated by their Government, turned against each other by unfortunate circumstances that keep reproducing themselves time and time again. The differences are obvious immediately after crossing the border. Did you know that, in Finland's schools, every child matters?

❧ III ❦

Right after the Savonlinna opera, I went to have a second series of discussions with Foerster Hadley Krupp and Dave Gutman, gods of Philadelphia start-ups. I remember how open heartedly and enthusiastically I went to these meetings.

I measure my important appearances by my wardrobe. This time, I was wearing the Finnish dress. The last time I sat among this group of entrepreneurs, I had not dreamed I would create a company. I had been in the middle of chemo and wearing my infamous blond wig. Of course, no one in the room knew anything about my cancer treatments. Only friends did. For consistency, I wore the wig again. I remember feeling good about my appearance. Maybe I never looked better in my life. And I believed so deeply in Dr. Dmitry's dendritic vaccine that I felt joy and inspiration.

My story must have been emotional. I painted the picture of a penniless Russian scientist creating a cancer vaccine in a cold room in a collapsing building through the impossibly difficult post-Soviet times. I heard, in my childhood, about a winter in besieged Leningrad where workers and school-children wore gloves and hats at factories and in schools, breathing out warm air visible in the frosty mist. This must have been something like the picture I painted.

The technology I was describing was, of course, powerful. Somebody mentioned Dendreon, a company that had been developing a dendritic vaccine for years. They were in the news because the FDA finally approved their treatment for prostate cancer. It was becoming clear that the technology Dr. Dmitry was mastering was valuable. A company that could develop it would have investors.

The groups from PSL agreed to work with the company. I was so happy. The work started shortly after the meeting and proceeded fast. As a result, we had a couple patents and an avid supporter, one of the best business law firms in Philadelphia.

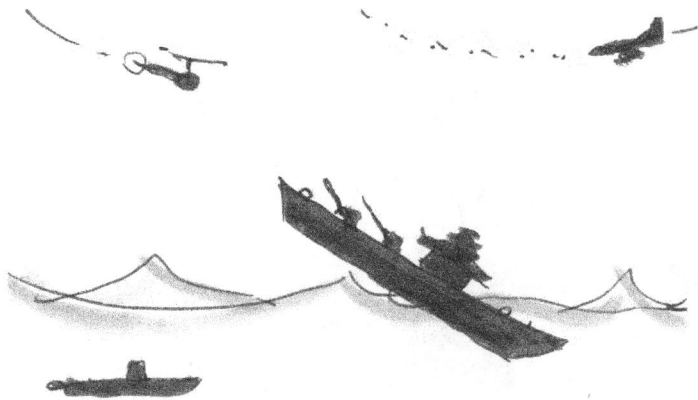

CHAPTER 48
Identity

I was bubbling with enthusiasm. The company was created, the documents drafted and signed. I was on schedule. As my Russian mentor, Iv Iv, kept saying: "Keep pushing." And I did. The next thing on the list was the web site. This is where we had so much fun. Of course, the best solution was to pay a marketing firm to do do it. The price for a well-thought out web site was $6-8 thousand. Cyrill yelled in horror, so I asked my friends Ken and Thomas to help out. OK then, I said, we'll do it. I wrote the code. I didn't like programming anymore, especially after the stroke, but suddenly it was structurally sound and ready for the images and concept. We considered a variety of concepts.

"Health... Let's show happy faces..."

"No, no. Happy faces are on every pharma company's web site..."

"True... But so what? Don't you want to be just like every other pharma company?"

"Hmm... I don't know..."

Ken would send me and Thomas the images of happy old people, looking at the horizon, playing tennis, sun-lit, at the beach, walking, with their grandchildren, happily old, never dying. A day later, everybody decides happy faces are boring.

"No... It's boring. This is not it. I thought I was gonna die, it is scary, and it should be scary, because it is life and death..." Ken said.

I recalled how I felt back then. Devastated. Scared. Dying. Counting time. I saw death.

"It's death. It is the fear of not living here anymore. Imagining your children grow up without you... it should be shocking. Like wake up and do something for yourself," he insisted.

"You want to be disturbing?"

"Yes, I want to tell people that they don't have to die. They have to be scared of death."

"But having death on the website... Let me think about it."

Then the next day Ken would send us Death: St. George the Dragon Slayer... Warriors on the horses... Knights in armor... Russian army fighting the Teutonic knights in the movie, what movie, *Alexander Nevsky, oh, that, I hate that, why, the score is Prokofiev's, yeah, perhaps, Its Russian too. Stalin's favorite...* Nah. I hated it, because it was Stalin's favorite and a patriotic stint demonstrating to everybody the superiority of a Russian tyrant. True, Dr. Dmitry is Russian and he demonstrated the superiority over all American treatments for me, for my life, for everything that mattered to me. But to glorify Stalin is something I could never do. I am a descendant of political jailbirds, murdered priests, hiding Jews.

We looked at the Death concept for a couple of days. Then we looked at Alexander Nevsky... Death and salvation…"Eureka!" Ken shouted in an email. He sent us the stills from the Hitchcock's "The Life Boat."

"Maybe, maybe," we said. But it was clear that the main theme was done. Immunotherapy was a lifeboat. I created the prototype and did a mini-survey among my friendly creatives. Then we sat down with Thomas to describe in detail what immunotherapy is. Thomas is a graphic designer, and for him T-cells meant nothing. I had to make it clear to him, first, what it was all about: the immune system, how it works and why, and how immunotherapy treatment stimulates it to repairs itself.

"Because it is a defense."

"Okay."

"A defense system that malfunctioned."

That was a pretty high level explanation.

"Then there are the details: the T-cells kill the enemy."

I could almost see how the defense system vocabulary was bubbling in Thomas' head.

"OK, who is the enemy?"

"Cancer cells."

"But how do they know who to kill?"

"Good question. They have something wrong with them and it is on their surface like the enemy flag. The antigen."

Men thinking about war become little boys. Thomas pulled out a childhood drawing of ships firing, people running, tanks and rockets.

"This makes sense," he said.

"But wait. It's not so simple," I tried to get into the details of my lifeboat equipment. Thomas was already nervously trying to sketch something on his drawing paper.

"There are dendritic cells. They are like spies."

"Oh! Spies!"

"Spies that let the soldiers know who is the enemy."

"What soldiers?"

"The T-killer cells of the immune system. They kill. They dissolve enemy cells, the cancer cells, the ones that were pointed out to them as the enemy. The cancer with the flag of an antigen."

"Let's go over this again. The spies. The immune system, a defense system, but sinking, not doing the job, not fighting the enemy."

Within a couple days, Thomas came up with a series of drawings: scenes of gradual recovery of the defense system and the destruction of the enemy. Submarines, rockets, and victory. It was a perfect reference to a Russian science too, in a mind of every American a connection to a powerful armor. It was all there: Russia, the mystery of the powerful enemy, the sophistication of technology. With this mysterious web site, we marketed Dr. Dmitry's dendritic vaccine without giving away any details. Cyrill shrugged his shoulders. Nothing could please him. He also stopped sending me money.

"Just keep pushing it," Iv Iv kept saying. "Just keep pushing."

The next step in finding a big investor to do clinical trials was to polish the business plan. I started to gather a formal team of scientific advisors. There is a lot of Big Pharma in Philadelphia and many pharma startups. The community was very welcoming and the path ahead became clearer. It was an exciting time for the American side of the company.

I want to sing a tribute to all of my board members: to all of you who spent countless hours with me and went through countless emails, I am so thankful for your trust. I want to thank you for your belief in immunotherapy and in Dr. Dmitry's brave scientific mind.

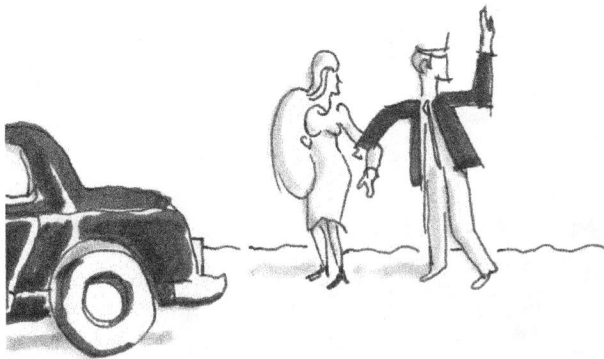

CHAPTER 49
The Warning

I met a French man at one of the Pharma conferences in Saint-Petersburg.

"What? You started a company with the Russian guys?" He seemed concerned.

"Yeah, but this is not what you think, they are all right!"

"All Russian businessmen play the same game."

"Oh no, my investor almost died from Big Infectious C…"

"And?"

"And now he wants to cure the world."

"Let me tell you, naïve American woman, what is gonna happen to you."

"No no, you don't understand. We are in the same boat. The other partner was cured too."

"Listen to me. What happened to me several times was this. You suggest a way forward. They say: 'No. You are crazy. It's not gonna work.'"

"Sure, that happened to me too."

"Fine. Let me continue. So they 'allow' you to do your plan that they called crazy. You work your ass off and it works out. You know how it goes."

"Sure," I kept nodding with reluctance.

"So, you had the idea, you made the plan, you do everything yourself, they promise you money, they put out a little bit but keep telling you it's not gonna work and that you have nothing of value. Then, when you start to see results, they say 'Oh by the way, we're gonna take this thing.' They don't even know what to do next, unless you shared your plan with them, which you did because you thought you were together in one boat."

"But... but he was cured, and I was cured, it..." I mumbled something with a fading objection.

"So if you let me finish."

"Go ahead, please."

"They will hijack your idea, push you out, and derail the whole thing because—and this is the worst part—they don't know how to do it."

"What did you do?"

"Learn your lesson and move on. The world is big. Start something else with different people, smarter now. You have to know what these people are about. They are suicidal but this instinct is stronger than anything for them. They can't change it, they want to be alone and get rid of everybody."

"Are you sure?" I still refused to let go.

"Am I sure? Listen baby. They will suck our blood out your

poor body. They did it to me, and I had to leave. And start another venture."

"I bet not in Russia, then?"

"Why not? I love Russia."

It did not make sense. He was screwed but he came back.

"With the new knowledge baby. With the tough love. Be tough, girl."

Then a beautiful, well groomed woman came up to him. I could tell she was smart.

"Okay, we've got to go." He smiled sadly at me.

"Nice meeting you..."

They left like two beautiful butterflies, iridescent and shining—was the woman wearing diamonds against her perfect skin?—in the aura of content and calm of a couple in peace with each other and the world. Did I imagine she was wearing a fur coat, or was it real?

Now I understood why this French gentleman stayed in Russia. His woman was first class. My predicament was different, there were no first class men rushing toward me like this classy woman must have rushed toward this savvy French businessman. I imagined her mildly desperate in the desert of Russia, where she could not possibly get a classy man from the spoiled, cruel and dominating bunch of alpha-s, or from the oppressed and weak beta-s, those two classes into which Russia now divides its men.

CHAPTER 50
Crazy

I was not ready for the sharks, I must admit. I was not ready for the obvious. Cyrill stopped answering my emails and, when I saw him at our meetings, he acted as if he was slightly annoyed with anything I said. His pervasive cynicism was becoming the norm. Anything I said would be met with a stare and he invited Dr. Dmitry to be stunned along with him. Cyrill had constructed a stage upon which he played the part of psychiatric doctor demonstrating the craziness of a patient (me) to his audience (Dr Dmitry).

Dr. Dmitry was becoming nervous. On one hand, he did not have any objections to my numerous proposals on how to move forward. On the other, he brought Cyrill in specifically as a business man, and now he had to obey him. He was trying to make peace, as much as he could. Cyrill would not talk to me and would not listen to me, and I was not about to let him call me crazy. Dr Dmitry found the situation annoying. "Anya, just let him drive, why are you struggling?" He did not know what to do. He was very unhappy with the way two people he had saved suddenly became the worst enemies, circling the medicine that had saved them.

Dr. Dmitry was very involved in his lab. All these arguments were distracting him from his beloved vaccine, his conversation with God. He was losing interest in the idea of patents and business arrangements. He could cure people; that was all that he cared about.

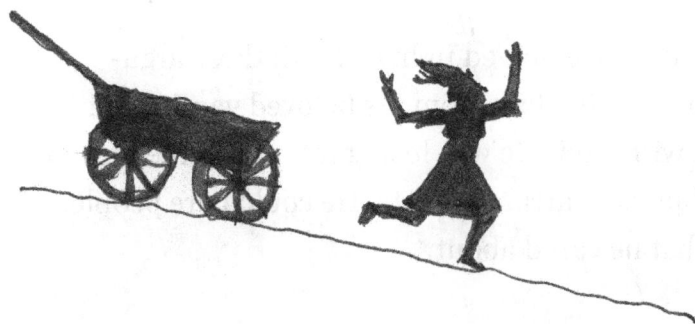

CHAPTER 51

More is More

*"Forgiveness is giving up all hope of having had
a better past." - Anne Lamott*

✷ I ✷

"Anya," Dr. Dmitry would say over and over again. "Please
let them drive if they want."

"But where are they driving?"

"It does not matter. Just let them drive."

"Fine," Iv Iv advised. "Let them drive."

Cyrill continued to play his game of a doctor despising his
female patient, a powerful lunatic from America, who would
be easy to destroy if she had not used his money to hire so
many lawyers. I was getting tired of the power struggle.

"Okay," I said. "If they want to drive, they can go ahead."

Cyrill started his driving. He drove to Maxim, my first
lawyer, who wrote our original agreement and saw our first
application through to become our first granted patent.
Cyrill yelled at him so passionately that Maxim became
really scared. He called me and his voice shivered.

Cyrill's next act was to drive to the other lawyers who were
working for us in Saint Petersburg and yell at them, too.

They started to wonder what was going on. They understood that I had to succumb under the threats, something that my American side never understood. The Saint Petersburg lawyers remembered Russia's bloody 90's when business disputes left corpses. Their advice was always to run away from threats. Some of them were scared for me. This is what life had taught them. I am surprised I did not succumb to the pressure, but I had been forced to give up so many times before, the notion of yet another abandonment of the fruits of my labor was simply not an option that time. Even the threat of death from Cyrill's 90's-style business toolbox did not make me run away. I am still surprised by myself, actually.

"The world is big," a lot of people in Saint Petersburg would say. "The ocean is blue. Swim away and start a new life."

☆ II ☆

A friend of mine told me a story about shoes. She was in Paris for the first time in her life outside of Russia. She had a little money and bought a pair of shoes. Alas, the shoes did not fit. She found this out after she had already paid for them. She tried to return the shoes to the store and get her money back. The clerk at the store refused.

"You already paid for them. We can exchange them..." the clerk would say.

"No. I want my money back," my friend repeated. "I just want my money back."

My position with Cyrill was kind of like that. I just could not leave my own ground, even though I knew it was becoming dangerous. I just stood there and said: "No. I am not a lunatic. I created this company. I created the patents. I am not getting lost just like that." Not only did Cyrill hijack the patent management, he forced Dr. Dmitry to abandon any other work he was doing with me.

Dr. Dmitry was not happy with my stubbornness. He seemed frightened for himself, not for me, and he was blaming me for my inability to work something out with Cyrill.

What could that something be? Just let them drive? Aren't they already driving?

I wrote a proposal with the help of a wonderful Russian lawyer.

"Don't act against your own interests," he would tell me many times. I think I had a tendency to give up too much, just to not be bothered. However, every time I gave in a bit and thought we could reach an agreement, Cyrill would write another proposal, asking for more. This battle was conceived to weaken the enemy, to cost her money, and to cost her time and motivation.

"Anya, you are too emotional," Dr. Dmitry would tell me many times.

This a typical argument a bully uses condescending when he is beating up his crying victim: "Hey girl. You are too emotional."

"What's wrong with being emotional? Can you do anything if you are not passionate about it?"

"Just too emotional."

I knew from my own life and from other people's that being emotional with your projects is the key to success. It felt like my life was being taken away from me. Dr. Dmitry gave it to me with one hand, and now Cyrill was taking it away. I started to question the worthiness of holding my ground. I was willing to negotiate, he was not. His final proposal was a natural progression of me giving up what he wanted to take. He demanded that I give all the shares in the company that I created to Dr. Dmitry, thinking that since I owe my life to him I would look very bad if I refused to do that. Also he proposed that all liability for the past, present and future would still be on me.

He also worked through my husband. It was the last straw in my marriage. Thanks Cyrill. You finally absolved me from any guilt towards poor Gosha, whose loyalty to you, a man, a school mate of the Leningrad Special Mathematical School number 239, happened to be stronger than his bond to me, his wife of sixteen years. Thank you, Cyrill, for making me strong over these three years by being such an obstacle in developing the Big Infectious C vaccine that could have helped so many people all over the world, because you wanted all the glory and money for yourself.

This is my tribute to you, Cyrill, thank you for teaching me so much about life. I hope to forget you soon. I pin you down in my imaginary butterfly collection, and add a little tag "Cyrill Rotkov, the Darwinian man: Eats human time and soul." I'll close the glass cover. I'll put the case on the shelf and take it out for my great-grand children.

❧ III ❧

The American lawyers did not understand.

"Why did you have to give him anything when he did not meet his contractual obligations?" they would ask.

Everybody was in awe and disbelief. I felt horrible. I felt that I failed all those people who helped me on both sides of the Atlantic, those who worked without being paid, believing in the great cause. They had been willing to donate their time to support the lifesaving vaccine invented by a penniless Russian Scientist. Members of the Scientific Board, my friends, had spent endless hours discussing strategy with me. I had met so many great people at all those pharma meetings: the best lawyers, who were not paid, the veterans of the biotech start-ups, those who specialized in clinical trials, lawyers, CEOs, fund managers, all in vain.

I was not prepared for such an outcome. I could not believe the lies that were circulated, the blame that went on, the search for mistakes and the desire to push me out and find me guilty. This was extremely unfair, unexpectedly terrible, and as result extremely stressful. The drama with Cyrill had gone on too long. My friends became concerned about the stress that could negatively affect my health.

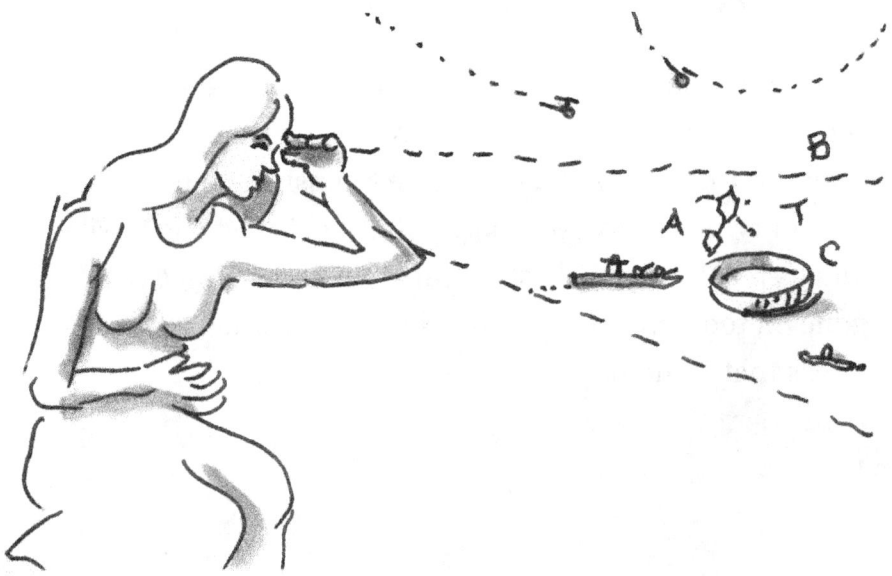

CHAPTER 52

The Cure for Cancer

"Hey," said my genius cellular biologist friend, "Come help me start a company on cancer stem cells."

I desperately needed distraction and a new positive direction. Cancer stem cells were to become my next preoccupation. Even as my friend, David Vausse, began to educate me on cancer stem cells, though, I found I still mourned the company I'd failed to launch. Okay, I thought, *Bye–bye immunotherapy.* But, it just so happened that my work with immunotherapy would prove vital in this next stage of my business life.

◆ I ◆

There is hope for us in stem cell research. Since stem cells can become nerve cells, they could theoretically be used to repair nerve damage and cure paralysis. Not all stem cells are the controversial embryonic stem cells taken from an embryo. Adult stem cells circulate in our bodies. They rush to the site of a scratch and substitute themselves for injured skin cells, eventually transforming into skin cells. This is possible because stem cells are undeveloped and therefore non-differentiated. When the right signal comes, they begin development, specializing, becoming whatever type of differentiated cell is needed. Multipotent stem cells can only become one particular type of cell. Pluripotent stem cells can become any type of cell.

Cancer cells with the abilities of pluripotent adult stem cells are a newly discovered player in the process of metastasis. My cell biologist friend told me all these horrible stories about the inventive tricks of cancer stem cells and how important they are in the formation of metastasis. Chemotherapy actually selectively adapts cells to make them drug resistant. Stem cells hide from chemotherapy. They move to different sites and try to become the surrounding tissue. They anchor to this other tissue and become a metastasis. Ninety percent of people who die from cancer actually die from metastasis, not from the primary tumor. Restricting the ability of cancer cells to metastasize should be the cure for cancer. It was fascinating and wonderful. I felt we were on the front line of an important frontier.

Something keeps the cells of the body committed to their specializations. The differentiated cells that compose our muscles, bones and organs can theoretically de-differentiate, like a professional who goes back to college to pursue a new field of study. The same mechanisms work when stem cells mutate and become cancerous, or when a cancerous cell de-differentiates and becomes multipotent or pluripotent. A couple of companies have sprung up, trying to find drugs that can kill these cancerous stem cells. They discovered, however, that killing one batch of cancerous stem cells doesn't stop others from de-differentiating.

All cells, it appears, cycle between different stages of development and, in the case of cancer, they accumulate mutations at different points of this interrupted, imperfect cycle. Cancer cells that differentiated at point A can become undifferentiated, returning to pluripotency at point B. Can a combination of drugs stop the growth of all these kinds of cells at all possible stations in their journey and with all possible mutations that they manage to accumulate? How do you target an enemy that continuously shape-shifts, mutates, divides?

✦ II ✦

Then it occurred to me. It was a stroke of insight. Immunotherapy introduces a constant surveillance mechanism: immune system cells multiply and hunt cancer cells day and night. Cancer cells are targeted at every stage of development, even in dormancy, as well as in every kind of tissue.

My God. The cells we'd used as an antigen had been from the fluid removed from my lungs. The malignancies found in that fluid would have been cancerous stem cells. The dendritic cells in the vaccine had functioned naturally, telling my immune system to target the cells in the antigen. However, my antigen included not only cancerous cells, but cancerous stem cells. I could hardly breathe. I had, in effect, done an anti-metastatic vaccine!

I am living proof of what really could be the conclusive cure for cancer.

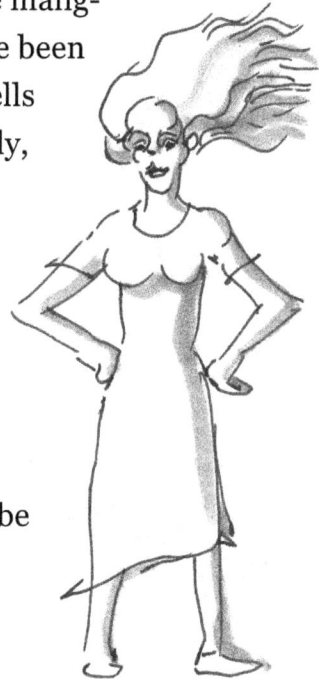

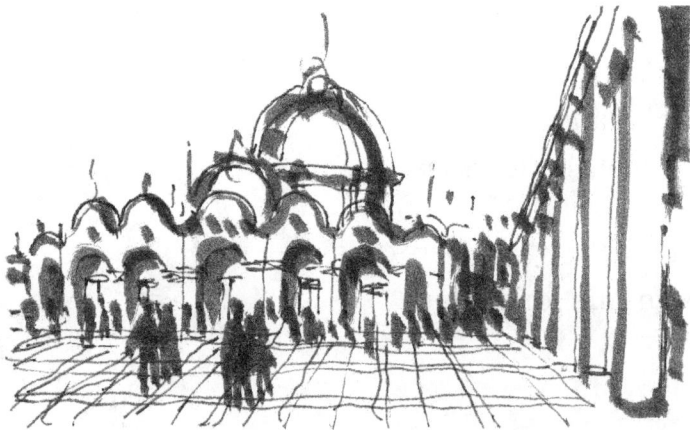

Conclusion:
The Meaning of Life

————◆•◅ɜ•६•◆————

A little, thinking girl switches off the street whoosh, the night sounds, her parents' distant murmurs, from her bed. Under a blanket, in her own space, alone in the dark, she thinks: *Why am I me?* Then, a terrifying thought, *As soon as I know the answer, I will die!*

Then, as a woman, she asks herself: *Why live? For myself? For my children?* Please do not answer these questions. As I learned, they have only unsatisfying answers. Only time spent aware, feeling, living, matters in the end. Perhaps, sometimes, we feel the connection to the rest of the world, but then we come back under the blanket and are at peace again, in the dark, without time. I cannot comprehend this mystery: the mystery of me, just me, experiencing my own life, forever alone and only.

◅ **I** ६

My parents were everything, my entire world, when I was little. They wanted me to live. I knew it so well. I knew it because they would panic at the slightest fever: it could be a deadly disease! A fall from a bike might mean tetanus! An upset stomach after eating a spoiled meatball, a head injury after a fight with my cousin... Every time, and many more, my parents went pale. So, all my early thoughts about my own death were related to the desire not to upset my parents.

To them, my death would be such a disaster, such a griev-
ous loss. But, what would the loss of my life be to me? In
the moments before I fell asleep, in the dark vortex adjacent
to that secret self-knowledge I was sure would kill me, when
I would think about reaching out to part the curtain, I held
back. I could not stand the thought of hurting my parents
by even thinking of my own death. My fear was the shadow
of theirs. I felt I could not risk self-knowledge because it
seemed it would result in a criminal self-annihilation.

Death was a taboo subject, absolutely forbidden. Not only
did I know it was paramount that I not endanger myself,
but I knew I must never speak of death, never think of it,
never question the idea that it was plain bad. No reason was
ever given. Like any taboo, this one was a commandment,
a rule; a thought about death was a sin, an evil. I knew I
needed to live in order not to overwhelm my parents with
grief. I was supposed to live. I was supposed to want to live.
It was an imperative. I was supposed to live by all means.
This was the rule. I was supposed to be afraid of dying. This
is how we all are.

⇥ **II** ⇤

I was given a second chance: a great warning. I heard it.
Now, I try never to forget it. And, if I do forget, I remind
myself of the feeling of the urgency of life. Most of us don't
know why we really choose to live, don't know the meaning
of our own lives, because society tells us we are supposed to
live without answering the question: "Why live?"

It sounds like a question of the suicidally depressed or the irresponsibly apathetic, but really it's foundational. Once, my reason for living was "not to sadden my parents." Then it became "not to sadden my kids." But I don't want my life to rotate around fear of loss. I don't want to wake up morning after morning trying not to think of the secret question.

→ III ←

Nobel prize winner, Ralph Steinman, who coined the term "dendritic cells" in 1973, died of pancreatic cancer three days prior to receiving his reward. He had been administering a vaccine to himself for four years. Perhaps, if he had known about cancer stem cells, he would be alive today.

Although Dr. Steinman died at 68 from the disease he aspired to cure, his efforts were anything but in vain. In addition to his service to humanity, Dr. Steinman gave himself the gift of time. He lived to see weddings and grandchildren. Life is all about the time we have together.

→ IV ←

This is the only tangible happy ending I have: more time. I wish I could say that the vaccine against metastasis was already in clinical trials. I wish I could say that it had begun to inspire other research and new companies. What happened, you might ask? And why don't all cancer patients now have access to anti-metastatic vaccines?

I feel extremely guilty, Dear Reader. I should have tried harder. I should have thought less. I should have been more persuasive, more selfless. The truth of why my second company disbanded is hard to believe.

The words are written in the sky. What was said, now is. Did I know this ruthless and beautiful truth, as I raced toward the dreams in my heart? My quotidian ego whispered them in my ear: to make a lot of money, to retire to a castle in Italy... My ego was dreaming its traditional dreams... Aloud.

"All I want, when we are done making our vaccine," I told my dear scientists, "is to retire to an Italian estate. After we make all the vaccines and all the money," I said, "I want to go to Italy and write. I would live in Italy and write a book."

I don't really know why I had this dream, to be a lazy writer, an estate owner in a luxury of chaise lounges and leisure. Perhaps I inherited it from my grandfather who was an actor and a dandy and a rebel: this dream of a bourgeois existence. It was always waiting in the back of my head like instructions. Go to Italy. Write a book.

"What?" Such frivolous, whimsy appalled my partners. These scientists stared at me across the table in their kitchen, over a near-empty bottle of Pinot Grigio. They were outraged. I was trying to defend myself. I felt like a little baby Greek goddess devoured by her father titan Khronos. I loved my friends, they were like parents to me. *Oh My God! What have I done?*

They misunderstood. They thought I was only developing immunotherapy vaccines for money! The next day they called and said they were leaving the company. They couldn't believe I dreamed of Italy, of becoming a writer, of living a life of hedonism in the pellucid early evenings. They dreamed only of flasks and cells: this was the meaning of their lives. They judged me because it was not the meaning of mine.

It was all so profoundly depressing that I decided to connect with a friend and go to Italy, just to see the beauty of nature and human history blend in a way it does so perfectly there. At that moment, I had no idea that I would actually start a book the moment I arrived.

This is the story of how my words were written in the sky since I said "Italy" and "book" in the same sentence. The sky did not know that I wanted to get the company off the ground first, generate income and then go Italy and write a book. Since I omitted that part, I only got what I shared: Italy and the book. Be careful what you wish for, is the old adage. But I do, also, one day wish to launch an immuno-therapy vaccine.

⇥ V ⇤

Just recently, a friend told me about a preventive vaccine for women who, due to BRCA gene mutation, have an 80% chance of eventual breast cancer. I hope we can develop it soon! I continue to dream and to work on bringing antimeta-static vaccines to more people. I go to conferences and speak to scientists whose lives *are* their immunotherapy vaccines. Every time I thank the scientific audience for their efforts, I get the warmest gratitude, even though they are the ones who saved me. I am eager for my worlds to connect again: to be engaged, to be social, to be able not only to share a common goal but to share the future by working together.

I wish I could report my vaccine is already in clinical trials, but I am back at square one. Perhaps with this book I will change that. With this book in hand, I hope to construct a team of dedicated scientists, find an investor to finance the effort, and finally succeed in creating and providing immune vaccines for every body and every disease.

I write it in the sky.

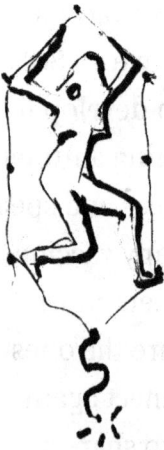

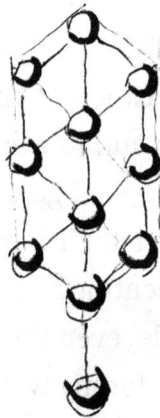

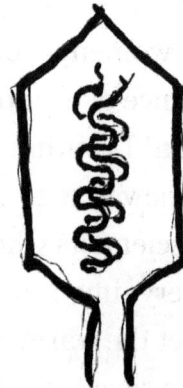

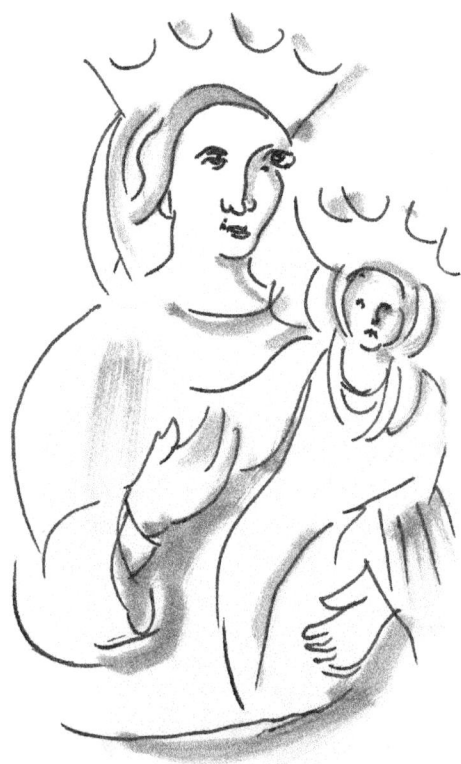

Epilogue:
Memory of Venice

Heavy memories destroy us, but the good memories are who we are. My memory of a memory of Venice... that we are walking, as in a dream, in the wrong direction, away from San Marco. We took the water bus, The *Vaporetto*, from our monastery. It was the only non-Venetian place in Venice: too ascetic and too new at the same time. The dream of an ideal Venice was patchy, and did not include certain shops and restaurants, and our room. But, the view from the canal was breath-taking and we forgot all our aesthetic disappointments when palazzo after palazzo opened up as the water bus carried the stunned crowd closer and closer to the Laguna and the infamous San Marco.

In this dream I said: "Here." And we stepped out from the boat. Perhaps it was becoming too beautiful. Perhaps I was getting nervous because we did not have the tickets. We turned to the right from the Grand Canal and kept walking through the very quiet residential neighborhoods with very simple houses so that, at times, they reminded me of the Italian neighborhoods in Philadelphia.

We were lost. There were canals, houses with boats in front, people living simple Venetian lives. Fondamenta Fornace. We looked like stupid tourists. Then we walked out to the open Laguna on another Fontamenta: ZattereaiSaloni. It is translated as "foundation," and it is a walking space along the canal. When I was a school girl in Leningrad, we would translate Saint Petersburg's "fondamenta" to "embankment." We were now on the Fondamente Zattereai Saloni overlooking Guideica Island with Palladio's cathedral, his only building in Venice.

"Hmm. Let's go this way," I said and we turned right again. It did not look like we were getting close to San Marco, and Olga was losing patience.

"Where are you going?" A man in his seventies asked us this in English.

"San Marco. Thank you for asking. How do you know we were lost?"

"The two beautiful and very tall ladies should be romantically lost in Venice."

We laughed.

"Of course two beautiful and very tall ladies are looking for San Marco?"

"Of course."

"This is in the opposite direction. Did I say this right?"

"Yes, of course."

"You mean I said that right?" he asked.

"Yes, yes. Why do you have doubts?"

"I am translating from Japanese. I am saying it in Japanese first and then I translate it into English."

"Oh wow."

"Yes, I lived in Japan for many years. I was a representative of Italy in Japan. Where are you from?"

We, of course, anticipated the question. The answer would differ depending on the circumstance, mostly on who was asking and how much complexity we would anticipate him to be able to handle. This old man seemed capable of a few twists.

"Russia and America at the same time," I said

We outlined, in a few sentences, that we were born in Russia but then lived in America, and that Olga will go back to Russia.

"I see. By the way, follow me and I will get you to San Marco. Follow me and I will get you there. I am used to helping out that way. I always helped my friend Katherine Hepburn when she got lost. If you've seen *Summer in Venice*?"

We turned around and started to walk alongside the old gentleman.

"Hmm. Did we hear that right? Your friend is Katherine Hepburn?"

"I told you right. Have you seen *Summer in Venice*? Oh did I say this right?" He mumbled something in a language that I assumed was Japanese. "Did I say this right?"

I did not remember if I had ever seen *Summer in Venice*, so I asked Olga behind his back. She indicated that she had. I now relied on her to continue the conversation.

"Yeah," he continued while we went on our walk along the Fondamenta in the wind. "I was the street urchin, a boy with the fishing rod. I was catching fish in the canal. I mean in the movie. It's windy today."

We were listening.

"I am from Giudecca. Look, it's the only Palladio in Venice."

We observed the Palladio from across the Canal

"I am from Giudecca. Nowadays all real Venetians live in Giudecca."

"I have a better idea for your time," he said, "Let me show you something. In the end, you can always go to Piazza San Marco, but this is more interesting."

Of course we did not mind to walk with such a guide.

"Let me show you the Church. Where did you get off?"

"Santa Maria Della Salute."

"Yeah. Did you go there? It's around the corner from here."

We did pass it on our way from the water bus, but paid no attention, concentrating instead on getting to the crowded San Marco. Now, we could look at nothing else. The church was so fabulously rich in décor that it was impossible to have a single thought. It was so overwhelming in its glory, so impossibly beautiful, that it made us feel tiny, our internal dramas a complete waste of time. Inside, it was sparse and much darker, even quieter. It was as if the bright Venetian sun had made a lot of beautiful noise on all those architectural details. Santa Maria Della Salute truly is one of the most perfect baroque buildings in the world.

"This church was built to spare Venice from the plague. And it did. A third of the population were dead."

He whispered something:"Did I say that right? In Japanese it would be... Did I say that right: the plague?"

"Yes."

"All these rats from the ships. Cargo? Is this the right word? The customs were right here, the next building."

The church had a circular plan and we walked its circumference, stepping on the contrasting dark and pale stones of the vortex floor. Titian hid in the darkness to our left, Veronese somewhere too. Madonna held the center, across from the entrance.

"This is the place where people pray for health."

We were standing in front of the Madonna.

"I will pray for your health," the Venetian gentleman said and turned inside for the prayer.

"Thank you," I said. "I will pray for yours too."

"Thank you, too," he said. "I need it."

We stood together and prayed.

❦ II ❦

How did he know I needed the prayer? I prayed for him, for Olga, for my children, my family, my friends, for Dr. Dmitry, for my friend Vika who introduced me to Natalya Nikolaevna who introduced me to Dr. Dmitry and yelled at me for good, for the pulmonologist who let me take my ascetic fluid, for the microbiologist who came up with the protocol for propagating my cells, for all those who donated money, for all those who organized my fundraiser, for all those who supported me. The circle expanded and expanded. I prayed for all the lawyers who helped me, for my business advisors who donated their time...

"Okay," the kindly guide interrupted the whirlpool of blessings. "Thank you ladies. When the church was built, the miracle happened and Venice was finally spared from the plague."

We continued walking the checkered circle.

"Maria della Salute... Madonna of Heath... Remember this moment. Do you promise you will remember this moment?"

We laughed: "We'll try!"

"No, no. I want you to remember this moment!"

"We'll remember, don't worry."

He became somewhat upset. "No, you don't understand."

We left the church and went for a walk. "I have an idea. Let me buy you something."

"Oh no, no."

"Accept the gift. You have to."

We were strolling down the narrow streets of Dorsudoro, knocking on doors of many merchants selling Venetian paraphernalia. Our guide did not like it there and we left. Finally he decided to stay on one street. He looked around the store.

"Prego," said the owner of the store in tender voice. I think our guide liked her and decided to shop in her store.

"I want to get them something to remember..." he must have said in Italian. "I told them about the movie *Summer in Venice*, I was a street boy in it."

"Prego," she said and let us look around. "Did you see the movie?"

"Yes," we said.

"Choose what you want," the guide said.

I decided I would get something inexpensive, just as a symbol. A small souvenir, so as to accept his gift. I was learning to accept gifts. I looked around. The usual touristy stuff: the carnival masks, the Murano glass figurines, postcards, albums, jewelry. I noticed a tray with huge glass rings for six euros. It seemed like a fine price, our Venetian guide would not certainly be hurt by it. I tried one ring on.

It was blue and deep in color, and huge.

"This," I said to the Guide. I was learning to accept the gift but still a little embarrassed, hurried, trying not to strike too much attention.

"No, no, no," the Guide said firmly. "This is not your size. But, the right size will look good on you."

He picked another ring. It was dark blue with a ribbon of white and gold alongside the curve of a glass drop: "Try it. I know it fits."

The Guide was right, it did fit. He paid for our gifts and we left the store, leaving the nice woman a little bit puzzled over the whole scene, I did not want her to think that we were using the old guy who wanted to be nice. He might have been there many times, with other tourists he picked up, giving them gifts.

We went to yet another store, a typical Venetian store, a dog wagging his tail, canvases in the back room, the gay customers. We walked around, the Guide bought me a little watercolor of the Doges palace, we left again. I gave this watercolor to Naomi when I got back.

"Oh," she said." I remember. "This is the Doges Palace."

"Thank you so much!" We shouted to the guide.

"No, no. Thank you for the time we spent together. I must get back."

I wanted to suggest a cup of coffee together, but for

whatever reason I did not. I was afraid that he might think we wanted something else from him, but we did not.

"Ciao," he said hurriedly. "Ciao. I have a surgery tomorrow, I did not tell you."

He started to walk away.

"Ciao," we said, stunned by his sudden departure. It seemed like he was not sure if he'd told us too much.

"Did I have a hat?" he looked frightened.

"No, you did not."

He turned the corner and disappeared down the narrow street.

I remember it all.

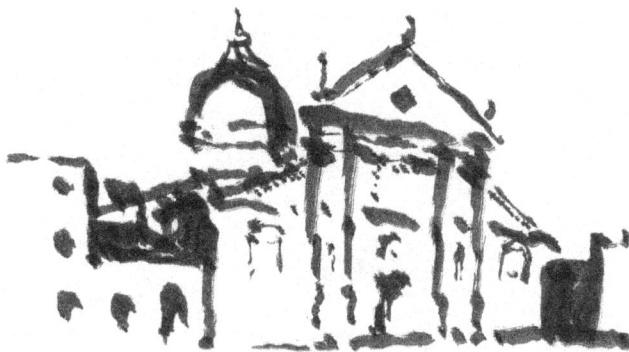

Appendix:
Letters to Susan Gubar

———————⟫•⟪———————

Dear Susan,

I just heard about your book and read a little on the web, and I am in a hurry to write to you.

I was diagnosed with stage 4 ovarian cancer in February 2009. I was very scared when an oncologist gave me 6 months to live. I was fortunate to have many biologist friends who connected me to a scientist in Russia. I was doing chemotherapy in the US and flying to Russia every month to receive my vaccine. The vaccine was the result of combination of several approaches and knowledge of several people, and I did not have any recurrences since then.

I am trying to get this treatment to more people. Fir which I started a couple of companies with these scientists, but getting money is difficult so far, without my story attached to the science of it. Basically it was immunotherapy with dendritic cells (something ubiquitous in clinical studies but nevertheless not readily available).

So I looked at raising money and getting this treatment to more women by writing a book or a blog, and I am half-way through it - it is both about the science of my treatment and about my experience during this journey.

It is not as eloquent as yours, but I believe it has a lot of merit for people who are going through the same thing in their lives, just as Solzhenitsyn's "Cancer Ward" was for me.

I hope that it will let people hear that treatments are available, and demand it from whoever are the gatekeepers of health.

Please write to me, because your book does exactly this -the irreverent demand for women's right to life in the 21st century science society.

I would like to talk to you more about ways to make this treatment possible - now.

Anna Gutkina

Dear Susan,

Thanks for your reply - I know how precious your time is. I guess especially after you wrote this book!

Before writing this response I was battling with the dilemma of writing prematurely: before I finish reading your wonderful book and run the risk to sound not fully informed about your

*situation, and before I finish polishing my book
to be ready for the exposure and critique, or
wait till I get to the end reading your of the book
and writing mine. If I waited and were ready,
I would then want to discuss that there are
parallels in your writing and in mine, we both
write about Kafka, and we both write about our
Jewish resilience and survival hunger, only my
Kafka is the Kafka of "Castle", not the "Process",
there would be many more things that I would
love to share, to be proud of, for you to critique,
etc, but.*

*I decided to write to you prematurely. Because
it is about vital information, something that
can save or prolong your life if you would like
to live. I think that even being as sad as you are
now, you should know - there is a possibility to
be treated with an immunotherapy vaccine at
the University of Pennsylvania. And it is totally
your desire to spend another couple years with
the people you love, or not to spend, to see your
grandchildren or not, to see your grad students
flourish or not, I understand. It is all about this
extra time. Immunotherapy adds no suffering to
your life, none. So there would not be a dilemma
of a life with suffering or the end of suffering and
dying from cancer. Your dilemma would be just
that- if you like to be here for more time.*

*Here is the link to immunotherapy trials at the
University of Pennsylvania:*

http://www.uphs.upenn.edu/obgyn/research/
ovarian_clinical.htm

They most likely will be dragging their feet and
find all kinds of reasons why they can't do it. But
I am willing to help you, as I know personally
some very good doctors, and I am thinking that
this safe and not so experimental (because it was
around for 20 years) therapy will improve their
stakes if you, Susan Gubar, would benefit
from it.

So please don't hang up and know that you may
help more people by granting your name to the
treatment that can really save women, like it
saved me. And I would not even suggest that
you read some chapters from my book but if
you want to get a biologist's perspective (vs an
English professor's) I could send you a link to it.

My best regards, and peace, and hope,

Anna

Bibliography

Cipolla, Carlo M and Freidrich Prinzig. "Italian plague of 1629–31." (n.d) Retreived 5 Oct, 2013. Wiki: http://en.wikipedia.org/wiki/Italian_plague_of_1629%E2%80%9331

Debeb, B. G., Lacerda, L., Xu, W., Larson, R., Solley, T., Atkinson, R., Sulman, E. P., Ueno, N. T., Krishnamurthy, S., Reuben, J. M., Buchholz, T. A. and Woodward, W. A. (2012). "Histone Deacetylase Inhibitors Stimulate Dedifferentiation of Human Breast Cancer Cells Through WNT/β-Catenin Signaling." *STEM CELLS*, 30:2366–2377. doi:10.1002/stem.1219

Fagone, Jason. *Has Carl June Found a Key to Fighting Cancer?* July 25, 2013. Web. http://www.phillymag.com/articles/carl-june-key-fighting-cancer/

Francis, Richard "Epigenetics: The Ultimate Mystery of Life." *Lamarck's Revenge*. 18 Aug 2011. Web. 26 Oct 2013.

Gessen, Masha. *Perfect Rigor: A Genius and the Mathematical Breakthrough of the Century.*
New York: Houghton Mifflin Harcourt, 2009. Print.

Gubar, Susan. *Memoir of a Debulked Woman: Enduring Ovarian Cancer.* 2012. Print.

Hay, Louise. "My Story." *The Light Connection.* December 2006. Web. 26 Oct 2013.

Androniki Kretsovali, Christiana Hadjimichael, and Nikolaos Charmpilas. "Histone Deacetylase Inhibitors in Cell Pluripotency, Differentiation, and Reprogramming," *Stem Cells International*, vol. 2012, Article ID 184154, 10 pages, 2012. doi:10.1155/2012/184154

Paulos, John Allen. "He Conquered the Conjecture." *The New York Review of Books*. 29 April 2010. Web. 26 Oct 2013.

Carol B. Ware, Linlin Wang, Brigham H. Mecham, LanlanShen, Angelique M. Nelson, Merav Bar, Deepak A. Lamba, Derek S. Dauphin, Brian Buckingham, BardiaAskari, Raymond Lim, Mu-neeshTewari, Stanley M. Gartler, Jean-Pierre Issa, Paul Pavlidis, ZhijunDuan, C. Anthony Blau. "Histone Deacetylase Inhibition Elicits an Evolutionarily Conserved Self-Renewal Program in Embryonic Stem Cells." *Stem Cell*.3 April 2009 Vol. 4, Issue 4, pp. 359-369. Web.

You can still attach your name to the great
cause of immunotherapy, a cure for cancer,
by funding further editions of this book.

To contact me and have your name published
in future editions, please contact us at
http://defusingcancerbomb.wordpress.com.

Thank you,
Anna

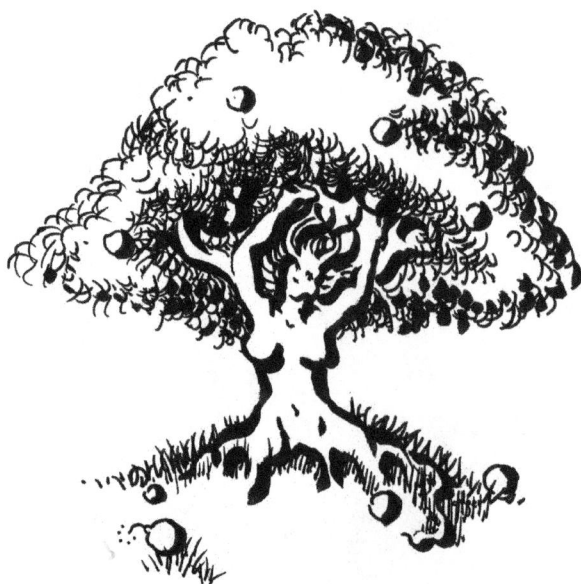

www.ingramcontent.com/pod-product-compliance
Lightning Source LLC
Chambersburg PA
CBHW081356270326
41930CB00015B/3317

* 9 7 8 0 6 1 5 9 6 4 5 4 6 *